OCCUPATIONAL THERAPY

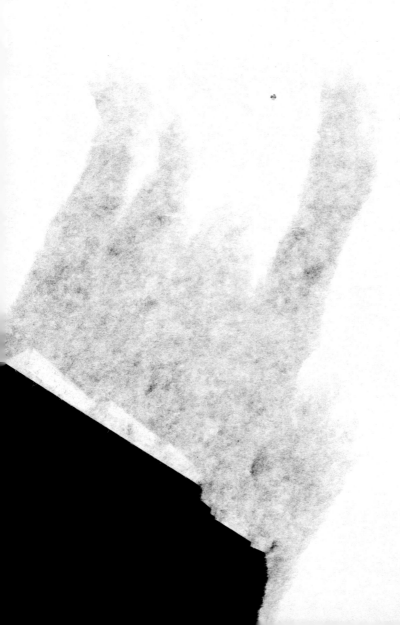

OCCUPATIONAL THERAPY

An emerging profession in health care

Report of a Commission of Inquiry
(Louis Blom-Cooper QC, Chairman)

Foreword by
HRH The Princess Royal

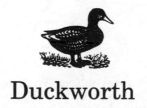

Duckworth

Second impression 1990

First published in 1989 by
Gerald Duckworth & Co Ltd
The Old Piano Factory
43 Gloucester Crescent London NW1 7DY

ISBN 0 7156 2330 3 (cased)
ISBN 0 7156 2331 1 (paper)

Photoset in North Wales by
Derek Doyle & Associates, Mold, Clwyd.
Printed in Great Britain by
Billing & Sons Ltd, Worcester.

Contents

The Department of Health were invited to send an observer to meetings and Mr John Rogers was nominated.

The College is grateful for the support of the King Edward VII Hospital Fund and the Nuffield Provincial Hospitals Trust.

BUCKINGHAM PALACE

In these days when more and more hospital patients convalesce at home and there is greater and greater pressure on institutional resources, the role of occupational therapy is becoming increasingly important.

Occupational therapy is still too often associated in the public mind with basket-making. In fact it has been revolutionised in recent years, along with all other medical facilities, and its members provide a wide range of caring and rehabilitation services within the community. One can hardly exaggerate the value of the work in restoring patients' ability to return to paid employment and regain personal autonomy and independence.

This excellent report is the first attempt to evaluate the profession as a whole. Its analysis of problems, and recommendations for future developments, are essential reading for all who care for our health services.

Anne

OCCUPATIONAL THERAPISTS MANPOWER COMMISSION

MEMBERS

Professor Eva Alberman

Mr Louis Blom-Cooper QC
Chairman

Sir Graham Hills

Professor Margot Jefferys

Mrs Patricia Marshall

Miss Mary Mason

Mr Hugh Pierce

Dr Douglas Price

Mr Brian Roycroft

Professor Philip Seager

Mr Peter Wood

Professor Andrew Young

Preface

At the end of 1987 the College of Occupational Therapists decided to set up an independent body to review and report on the present state of occupational therapy in the United Kingdom and its future role. The Commission of Inquiry (whose membership appears in Appendix A) was duly set up and given the following terms of reference:

> To review the existing activities and future demands upon, and the resources available to, the profession of occupational therapy, having regard to the social, demographic and epidemiological trends into the twenty-first century, and to report with recommendations.

The evident intention of the College in consigning the task of review to an independent body was not just to indulge in a piece of window-dressing. It was a serious move away from the stereotyped, internal review that organisations traditionally establish to ensure that their vested interests are well protected. From the outset the Commission was conscious that it was embarking upon its task in extraordinary circumstances. If not unique, it is, in the experience of all the members of the Commission, unusual for a professional association voluntarily and at considerable cost to expose its present and past activities, and its future existence, to the scrutiny of a group of people from disparate disciplines.

Preface

Throughout the Commission's deliberations the independence of the inquiry was scrupulously observed by the officers of the College, and none of the members had his or her objective judgment compromised.

At the request of the Commission, the Chairman and/or Secretary to the College attended all meetings in the capacity of observers. This enabled the Commission to obtain instantaneous information and assistance which greatly speeded up its discussions and deliberations. The Department of Health and Social Security (as it was throughout the earlier part of the work) likewise provided an observer. We are grateful to Mr John Rodgers for his helpful guidance. We met on eight occasions in 1988: 7 January (in London), 19 February (in Manchester) 14 April (at the College's AGM in Warwick), 19 May, 15 July, 1 September and 14 December (all in London). We met for a week-end in Edinburgh from 28-30 October, and finally on 12 June 1989 to approve and sign the report. The report was presented at the College's Annual meeting in Glasgow on 30 June 1989. We met some occupational therapists at their annual conference in Warwick and visited others in various parts of the country. (These visits are listed in Appendix A.) The persons and organisations who gave written and oral evidence are also listed in Appendix A.

We are grateful to Miss Caroline Riddell who, with the administrative back-up of the College staff, supplied all the necessary secretarial assistance with supreme efficiency and cheerfulness.

1

The Backcloth

Changing health needs and health services: the context

The dilemmas facing the profession of occupational therapy today have to be understood and resolved against the backcloth of the truly revolutionary changes that have taken place, and are continuing to take place, in the demographic and health profiles of the British population during the twentieth century. One set of stark statistical facts tells a compelling story. At the turn of the century only one in twenty people were over the age of 65; in 1989, the figure is one in six; and by the end of the century the very old – those aged 85 and over – will be about a million in a population of just under sixty million.

This major demographic shift is both the cause and the effect of the similarly revolutionary changes that have taken place in health needs, and consequently in the nature and volume of health service work. In the early years of the century medicine had little to offer adults who fell ill or were seriously injured. Its successes lay largely in public health measures designed to save infant and child lives by preventing infectious diseases to which the young were particularly vulnerable. Palliative measures designed to alleviate suffering rather than effect cures were carried out almost exclusively by two occupational groups – medical practitioners (the majority, general family doctors) and nurses working in hospitals and homes. Given widespread poverty, many people did not have ready access even to these two sources of support.

By mid-century the efficacy of medicine, both curative and preventive, had taken a significant leap forward. Previously, greater longevity had depended for the most part on improvements in nutrition and personal hygiene and relied on public health measures to make the human environment safer. From the late 1930s, however, pharmacological discoveries in the form of vaccines and antibiotics made it possible for infectious diseases to be either prevented or treated. Tuberculosis and poliomyelitis, which previously had killed or maimed, were brought under control, if not eliminated. In the hospitals technological innovations revolutionised or made possible new diagnostic and surgical procedures. The simple structure of health services personnel, composed almost exclusively of doctors and nurses, evolved rapidly into a complex of inter-dependent professions, each of which had a specific expertise to offer in the services now available to the sick. Through the National Health Service, successive governments have, moreover, accepted a commitment to make such services available free of charge to all in need of them.

The sequential effects of these changes in the health and demographic profile of the nation are also great. Not only have they created a demand for new kinds of expertise within the hospital sector of the National Health Service: they have also emphasised the need to develop domiciliary services which will allow increasing numbers of older, frailer people to live in peace and dignity in their own homes or in sheltered non-hospital environments for the length of their natural lives. In short, on both humanitarian and economic grounds, the need to provide caring and rehabilitation services in the community rather than in institutions is becoming ever more pressing.

Occupational therapy: a submerged profession?

Occupational therapy was one of the health professions to emerge in the years before the Second World War and to establish itself as supplying an indispensable service in its wake. What is occupational therapy? What professional work is done by those called occupational therapists? A brief account of the origins and subsequent history of the profession is essential to an understanding of at least some of the dilemmas which face it today.

Unlike radiography and medical laboratory work, occupational therapy did not develop primarily to enable medicine to exploit new technologies: it developed when it became possible to save the lives of those who would in earlier times have died. With this increased ability there was a growing awareness that the job of restoring individuals to health and maximising their functional capacity was not completed by the physician, the surgeon or even the bed-side nurse exercising their various skills. Many hospitalised patients who had survived invasive surgical or medical procedures were nevertheless listless and pessimistic about the future pattern of their lives. They often lacked the motivation even to leave the hospital, where at least they were sheltered from the realities of a possibly hostile world. In the world outside hospital they needed to be given sympathy, advice and practical assistance if they were to regain the skills required for them to function adequately in paid employment or domestic tasks – in short to establish as much personal autonomy and independence as possible. The health service needed to develop a rehabilitation thrust as an integral part of its therapeutic purpose.

Slowly it dawned on the few, dotted throughout the services, who were being employed to proffer such support to patients, that a new approach was required. These few were acutely aware that they themselves, by professional training, had to acquire a systematic body of knowledge and skills. It could not be given satisfactorily by amateur, self-taught well-wishers.

We examined several of the definitions of occupational therapy currently found in textbooks and dictionaries as well as the definition used by the College of Occupational Therapists. The College defines occupational therapy tersely as 'the treatment of physical and psychiatric conditions through specific activities in order to help people reach their maximum level of function and independence in all aspects of daily life'. While recognising that the activities of the occupational therapist may indeed be very varied, we found this definition and the others we examined too broad and unfocused to be useful as a description of the role. Feeling that an accurate definition was important for the future of the profession, however, we coined the following definition and recommended that the College adopt it:

Occupational therapy is the assessment and treatment, in conjunction and collaboration with other professional workers in the health and social services, of people of all ages with physical and mental health problems, through specifically selected and graded activities, in order to help them reach their maximum level of functioning and independence in all aspects of daily life, which include their personal independence, employment, social, recreational and leisure pursuits and their inter-personal relationships.

1. The Backcloth

In addition, for purposes of providing a general description, short of definition, we offer the following:

Occupational therapy is the exercise of skill, care and judgment in assessing the degree of a person's mental disorder or physical disability, and treating such a person accordingly, by selecting and utilising appropriate activities of that person's normal pattern of life.

Such activities may be modified or applied to the defined problem of either the individual with the specific disorder or disability, or the group to which that individual belongs.

The activities, modified or unmodified, are designed to achieve progress towards the attainment of maximum independence for the individual in the appropriate environment.

To perform these activities the core knowledge and skills required by the qualified occupational therapist can be roughly categorised under the following four main headings:

(1) Knowledge of the intelligence, physical strength, dexterity and personality attributes required to perform the tasks associated with a whole gamut of paid and unpaid occupations and valued leisure pursuits.

(2) The professional skill to assess the potentialities and limitations of the physical and human environments to which patients have to adjust and to judge how far these environments could be modified and at what cost to meet individual needs.

(3) Pedagogic skills required, first to teach people how to acquire or restore their maximum functional capacity, and second to supervise and encourage technically trained instructors and unqualified assistants in their tasks of implementing and monitoring therapeutic recommendations.

(4) The psychological knowledge and skills to deal with anxiety, depression and mood swings, which are the frequent aftermath of serious threats to health or of continuing disability, and to motivate, or remotivate, those with temporary or persistent disabilities to achieve their maximum functional capacity.

These four headings, elaborated in the detailed curricula of the schools of occupational therapy, became in essence the core knowledge and skills possessed by those described as occupational therapists. While some of the elements of their work may also lie within the competence of other professional groups, especially in the proliferating field of rehabilitation occupations in both hospital and community services, no other professional group can lay claim to the specific combination of knowledge and skills.

It has nevertheless proved difficult to eliminate an outdated image of occupational therapy – an image conjured up in the minds of the general public and, at times, by fellow health professionals. This image was neatly paraphrased in a recent article by a senior nurse in a mental hospital who expected, when placed in an occupational therapy department during training, that 'it meant the probability of 10 weeks watching occupational therapists direct clients into making wicker baskets and knitting squares for blankets! Alternatively, it could involve working in the hospital's successful market garden.'

A decade earlier the Chairman of the Social Services Committee of the Association of County Councils, while acknowledging the invaluable help given to handicapped people by occupational therapists and anxious to ensure a sound future for them in local authority social service departments, was constrained to describe them as belonging to 'something of a submerged profession'.

Some of the evidence we obtained during the course of our inquiry confirmed the persistence of outdated stereotypes of what the profession's work entailed in sharp distinction to the activities in which its members were actually engaged. Such stereotypes are undoubtedly a handicap to a proper regard for the status of the profession and an appreciation of the value of the work actually performed by occupational therapists. So much so indeed that we felt that the very title 'occupational therapy' could partially account for its remaining, despite a substantial growth in its numbers and far-reaching tributes to the value of their contribution, a 'submerged' profession.

The College of Occupational Therapists had itself recently considered changing the profession's name and might have done so, had an acceptable alternative been readily available. We felt that the issue was important enough to warrant our own investigation of possible alternative titles. The likeliest candidate is 'ergotherapy'. This has the advantage of being used by some other countries to describe work in health and welfare services comparable to that done by occupational therapists here. It suffers from the disadvantage of linguistic association with ergonomics, which is defined as the study of the efficiency of persons in their working environment. In its link with the patient's work, however, it is not wide enough to encompass the ambit of rehabilitation. Moreover to use the name 'ergotherapy' would, in some people's eyes, be importing a recondite word into the English language. To some of us this is not a handicap. We recall that in the early 1960s the introduction of the word Ombudsman, to characterise someone who adjudicated on complaints against government administration, often produced a giggle at such an alien and weird

17

Scandinavian concept. Today Ombudsmanry permeates every facet of governmental administration, to the point where, in relation to central government administration, it is used in preference to the authorised, statutory title of Parliamentary Commissioner for Administration. The objection to 'ergotherapy' is that, unlike 'ombudsmanry', it is not introducing a new name to a novel aspect of social engineering, but is seeking to replace an established occupational designation in the field of health and welfare services.

In the event, we were unable to agree to a change to 'ergotherapy', or indeed to any other, so far unsuggested, title. Hence we make no specific recommendation for change. We nevertheless urge the College not to give up altogether the quest for an alternative.

The establishment and maintenance of professional identity and autonomy

The struggle to establish a self-governing profession with control over recruitment and education, as well as standards of work, has been a long one. Nor has it yet been entirely successful, in the sense that occupational therapists, in common with some of the other professions covered by the Professions Supplementary to Medicine Act (1960), do not yet have security of title, despite the possession of state registration. Contemporary and prospective changes in the management of the National Health Service and in the functions of local authority social service departments, and in the objectives of these services, have brought new challenges, if not threats, to the profession. The reasons for the long and continuing struggle to establish and maintain an autonomous profession with an undisputed and universally respected identity are various. We believe that it is useful to review them, if only briefly, because they still contribute to the problems facing the profession.

The first is the dominant position held by the medical profession in the division of labour in the health service, and the similar domination of the social work profession in the local authority domiciliary social services. If the professional objectives of occupational therapy appear to conflict with the authority of either of these two professions they are likely to meet resistance, as they did from medicine in the decade prior to the passage of the Professions Supplementary to Medicine Act (1960). In such circumstances professional advancement for occupational therapists depends on either courting the dominant profession to acquire its patronage or forming alliances with other professions, similarly placed, in order to try to erect a common platform.

A second, allied reason is the dependence of occupational therapists on doctors and social workers for access to their clients. Those who can benefit from the knowledge and skills of occupational therapists are not able, let alone likely, to approach them directly. Client-support for their claims through the market is therefore not forthcoming, as it is for some of the other occupations which live in the shadow of medicine.

A third reason is that, in so far as the public (and often other personnel in the health and social welfare services) are aware of the existence of occupational therapists, they frequently display (as noted above) a false and damaging stereotype of their function, derived unmodified from the very earliest preoccupations of do-gooding volunteers. They are identified as mainly there to encourage reluctant men and women to take up basket, or other craft, work. Alternatively they are seen as performing unskilled, 'commonsense' tasks which do not merit the prestige accorded to doctors. Qualification for medical practice is reckoned to require high intelligence and long training. Even nursing, which is popularly regarded as requiring angelic dedication in carrying out essentially distasteful work, is given an enhanced status.

A fourth related reason is the pronounced female composition of the profession – another characteristic it shares with other health service occupations. Those who take up the profession of occupational therapy are often regarded not only by the general public but also by service managers as merely filling a time-gap between school-leaving and child-bearing and child-rearing. While the pattern of employment for women has changed in the last fifty years, older perceptions of appropriate behaviour die hard and continue to influence the pecuniary and other rewards that can be derived from work in predominantly female occupations.

A fifth reason, of comparatively recent origin, stems from the new managerialism called for in the National Health Service and – to a lesser degree – in local government. The imposition of cash limits, and restricted resources, although ostensibly encouraging value for money in expenditure (something which might well rebound in favour of more – not less – occupational therapy), has inevitably raised issues of efficacy. Given the difficulty of measuring the outcomes of occupational therapy procedures, and the competition for resources from users of high technology, the professional activities of occupational therapists are likely to be seen as peripheral to the main medical and surgical objectives of cure. They may even be judged as luxuries which a financially squeezed health service can ill afford. Indeed the hunt may be on to find ways of substituting pseudo-occupational therapy, performed by other professional groups or by technical assistants with no qualification in occupational therapy as such, in poor substitution for the genuine article. There is even talk in responsible circles of ending the separate identity of the various professions within the general field of rehabilitation and creating a single profession with specialisms developing only after initial training.

Paradoxically, the danger of imposing such second-rate solutions to the problems, as seen from a management perspective, arises not from the failures but the manifest successes in the last two or three decades. As the next chapter shows in detail, the profession has expanded more than the other professions supplementary to medicine. Even the greatly increased numbers who have entered the services in the last two decades cannot meet the demand for qualified occupational therapists in both the National Health Service and local government departments. The professional body (the College of Occupational Therapists) has no reason whatsoever to blame itself for many of the problems it believes now assail the profession. The problems (as this report seeks to demonstrate) arise typically in situations where the demand for the services of an occupational group is increasing, not declining, and outstrips the supply. Increasing demand on the profession creates dilemmas for those in it. It calls for measures to achieve necessary changes in the internal organisation of professional departments, and in external relationships with other health and local authority service personnel. These changes, in turn, have implications for the recruitment, training and retraining of occupational therapists and their helpers. Succeeding chapters address these issues.

2

Facts and Figures

One of the first questions we set out to answer was whether the present number of occupational therapists was sufficient to meet the demand from the two major employing authorities – the National Health Service and the Social Service Departments of Local Government. Further questions followed automatically. If there was a shortfall in supply, how serious was it? Was it evenly distributed throughout the country and between the two employing authorities? Was it mainly in the basic grades of the profession, or did it extend to senior, supervisory posts? What would be required of the profession and the employers to bring the supply and demand into better balance in the future?

In trying to answer these questions we had available to us some routinely collected data from the Council for Professions Supplementary to Medicine (CPSM), which was established in 1960 and is responsible for the registration of seven professional groups, including occupational therapy.[1] It also had some estimates from the College of Occupational Therapists. Neither of these

[1] The other professions are: chiropodists, dietitians, medical laboratory technicians, physiotherapists, radiographers, and orthoptists. Remedial gymnasts, for which the CPSM was once responsible, have merged with the physiotherapists. Another profession of more recent origin in the field of rehabilitation, speech therapy, does not come under the aegis of the CPSM.

two sources, however, could answer all the questions we wished to put; so we conducted our own enquiry with a questionnaire to every occupational therapy department in the NHS and to all Local Authority Social Services Departments (including the Scottish and Northern Irish equivalents) asking them for information about their staffing at 31 March 1988.[2]

The demand for occupational therapists

The relationship between the demand for, and supply of, any professional group's services is not a straightforward calculation. It depends, in the first instance, on how demand is calculated. The number of available posts in occupational therapy in both the NHS and local government has not been reached as the result of the application of a generally agreed national policy norm of posts per head of the relevant population to be served. The number of posts in this profession has just 'growed', like Topsy. The growth reflects a variety of pressures exercised on employing authorities – the main ones being those of population-ageing and changing perceptions of the potentiality of rehabilitating patients of all sorts after hospitalisation. Such pressures, however, do not exist in a vacuum. In responding to them, employing authorities have to be mindful of alternative legitimate pressures on their limited resources, and also of the likely availability of trained occupational therapists. This last, in turn, depends upon the rate at which training establishments can attract recruits and respond to pressure to enlarge their facilities. The authorities, moreover, have to act within the constraints imposed by

[2] The response rate of NHS departments was 91% and of local authorities 74%. Appendix B Annexes 2 and 3 provide the overall findings of this survey.

existing agreements relating to salaries and conditions of work imposed on them by the rules and regulations of a large, bureaucratic public-sector enterprise.

One of our recommendations (see Chapter 7) is that pressure should be put on central government to set out norms for the number of occupational therapy posts which both major employing authorities should establish. In the absence of such norms, however, we had to accept that the numbers of *established* posts in the NHS and Local Authority Social Service Departments (LASS) for occupational therapists and their unqualified helpers and technical instructors constitute, very roughly, the current *demand* for occupational therapy.

Table 1 shows the number of *established* occupational therapy posts at the end of March 1988 in the 192 NHS District Health Authorities and 86 Local Authority Social Service Departments which responded to the Commission's enquiry. The NHS posts, but not those in the local authority sector, are given by grade and qualification. Since some posts are part-time, the second column provides figures adjusted to Whole Time Equivalent (WTE) posts. If the figures in this latter column are taken to represent the *real* demand for occupational therapy, the national picture at 31 March 1988 indicated a ratio of 0.27 WTE posts in the specialty per 1000 of the UK population. Within the NHS there were 77 posts for unqualified helpers for every 100 posts for qualified professionals.

In order to compare the demand for occupational therapists in the different regions of the UK, we related the WTE established posts in each region to that region's population, and gave the result as a figure per 1000. This exercise showed that nine regions had posts equal or close to the national average. Two regions, Trent and SW Thames, were well above the national average and two others, East Anglia and South Western, markedly so.

Table 1. Established posts for occupational therapists at 31 March 1988

Qualified OTs in NHS	*Posts*	*WTEs*
District OTs	173	169.1
Heads	1213	1167.3
Senior OTs	4149	3479.2
Basic grade OTs	1752	1623.4
Sub Total	**7287**	**6439.0**
Unqualified staff in NHS		
Helper TIs	1689	1406.7
Helpers	3225	2437.8
TIs	799	724.8
Therapists	217	162.9
Others	398	254.9
Sub Total	6328	49877.1
Total NHS (based on 91% response)	13615	11426.1
Total LASS (based on 74% response)	1922	1669.2

NW Thames was well below the national average, and the Northern and West Midland regions, as well as Scotland, were markedly so (see Appendix B, Table 2).

These regional differences in the demand for occupational therapy did not follow any readily detectable pattern. For example, there was no clear association between above- or below-average figures and the common north-south divide which marks the country in so many different ways. There was some slight evidence, however, to suggest that districts within regions where there was a school of occupational therapy were rather more likely to have a greater than average demand in the form of established posts; this would make sense, since schools would be eager to establish opportunities close to them for their students to observe the work of practitioners. Such a tendency, however, could not fully explain the overall regional differences.

We also considered the possibility that the NHS

regions with a below-average number of established WTE posts were compensated by the existence of above-average local authority establishments. Unfortunately, because of the variable response rate, and the lack of correspondence of the NHS and local authority administrative areas, this possibility could not be systematically explored. In one region, however, the Northern, it could. Adding together the NHS and LASS posts made no difference to the low league position of the region in regard to the ratio of OTs per 1000 population. If that experience can be generalised, it suggests that the differences in the number of posts cannot be accounted for by either an automatic or a deliberately engineered compensation between employing agencies.

Earlier, attention has been drawn to the importance of an ageing population in the need for an expansion of occupational therapy. The Commission's analysis of demand, therefore, also calculated the number of NHS WTE posts in the regions allocated to geriatrics per 1000 of the population aged 75+ (Appendix B, Table 7). The national average of 0.63 was well exceeded in Northern Ireland, Oxford, South Western, Yorkshire, East Anglia and Mersey; but all the Thames regions, with the exception of NW Thames, were well below it. There was not a sufficient match between this measure of demand of occupational therapy services and the more general one of OT posts of all kinds per 1000 of the population to suggest that systematic regional differences exist in the significance given to the ageing population in setting overall staffing levels for this occupation. There were also marked regional variations in the proportion of NHS posts allocated to different client groups besides the elderly. For example, one region had allocated 20.9% of its WTE posts to the mentally handicapped, while another had a mere 2.2%. That there should be such major differences of this kind is further evidence that little rational thought has been given to the overall requirements for occupational therapy in the health and welfare services.

One additional point needs to be made before considering how far the effective demand for occupational therapy is currently being met. It is that demand can be artificially reduced. The survey showed that this can be done in two ways. First, established posts can be abolished as a result either of lack of funding or of continuing failure to fill them. There was evidence in the Commission's survey that this had happened in the 12 months to 31 March 1988, during which time an admittedly small proportion of previously NHS established WTE posts (0.84%) had been permanently cut. A further 1.1% had been temporarily frozen. Corresponding figures for the local authority staff were fairly close: 0.12% of all WTE posts had been permanently cut and 1.4% temporarily frozen.

These points need to be borne in mind when considering whether the existing number of posts, coupled with a steady expansion in numbers of trained occupational therapists, comparable to that which has taken place in the last decade and a half, will be adequate to meet the standards of service which the profession believes the people of this country have a right to expect.

Meeting the demand

Our survey indicated that there were 1,149.6 NHS WTE funded posts unfilled at 31 March 1988 in the 192 districts which responded to the enquiry. To this must be added 221 equivalent posts in the 86 responding local authority departments. On a national scale these vacancies amounted to approximately 10.3% of funded posts in the NHS and 11.9% of LASS funded posts.

On a regional basis NHS vacancy rates varied from as little as 4.0% in Scotland to four times as many (16%) in the South East Thames region (Appendix B, Table 1). Once again there was no easily discernible pattern in these regional variations. For example, low vacancy rates were found in regions where the demand was low as well as in those where the demand was high. The Thames regions covering London and the home counties, however, had above average vacancies, while the rates in other parts of southern Britain were on the low side. Our enquiry also showed little variation in the vacancy rates for posts allocated to different client groups in the NHS. The lowest vacancy rates of around 8.5% were found in community services and acute surgery. The highest rate was in mental handicap (12.3%) followed by mental illness (10.5%) (Appendix B, Table 5). In the local authority sector functional allocation was assessed differently. Most posts were allocated to a broad category called 'adult physical handicap'. Not surprisingly, it was in this area that most vacancies also occurred.

While it was difficult to discern patterns in the regional distribution of unfilled vacancies, it soon became apparent that there were marked differences in the vacancy rates of various staff categories within the NHS. The contrast between overall vacancies for qualified and unqualified staff was stark. Sixteen per cent of WTE posts for qualified workers were vacant on 31 March 1988, compared with less than 3% of equivalent posts for the unqualified. Among the qualified, however, the vacancy rates produced a different picture. The grading structure is complex and, in the analysis, we decided to group grades into a smaller number of categories, ranked in order of seniority (Appendix B, Table 3). The results

29

were startling. Among the qualified, unfilled vacancies in the highest grades were low, amounting to less than 5.0% of funded WTE District OT posts. In the Basic grade, by contrast, vacancies totalled more than 25.0%, or over one in four. Indeed it was found that, while this key category, where newly qualified recruits normally enter the profession, contained roughly 25% of all WTE established posts for qualified staff, it accounted for over 40% of the total number of vacancies for qualified OTs. The intermediate categories of Head and Senior OT had approximately 10% and 15% vacancy rates respectively. Such a pattern of vacancies, as is discussed later, is the inevitable hallmark of a rapidly expanding occupational group at a comparatively early stage of its development.

Some measure of the seriousness of the national personnel shortfall can be gained by looking at the length of time posts have been vacant (Appendix B, Table 4). Information on this matter was not always available, but, when it was, it showed that 68.6% of NHS vacancies for qualified OTs and 40.4% of those for unqualified OT-allocated staff had been unfilled for three months or more. In the local authority sector the figure for all staff was 65.9%.

Reasons for vacancies and the shortage of qualified occupational therapists

To what can the substantial number of vacancies – most of them of considerable duration – be attributed? Is it merely a question of the number of new recruits to the profession failing to keep pace with the rate of creation of new posts in the NHS and local government, or are there other factors influencing the picture? For example, is there an excessive number of qualified individuals changing posts within the profession, which could lead to an exaggeration of the problem of overall shortfall? Alternatively, is there a pool of qualified potential workers who are not available for the employment which is on offer because they are engaged in other paid or unpaid occupations? The Commission's own survey did not allow it to answer all these questions as authoritatively as it would have wished. Nevertheless it and the data which it obtained from the CPSM throw some light on them.

First, it must be said that the rate of expansion of posts in the NHS and, in more recent years, in the local authority sector has been very great. We have no precise data on the growth in the posts established to work with different types of patient or client in the hospital or domiciliary setting in the recent past, but the greatest growth seems to have taken place in three areas – geriatrics, mental illness and mental handicap – which now absorb between them nearly two-thirds of the allocated established posts in the NHS. Although the expansion of posts has been accompanied by a phenomenal rate of expansion in the numbers of qualified occupational therapists in the last two decades – a rate which has exceeded those of all the other professions whose qualified

Table 2. Numbers in different professions registered with the CPSM

	1971	1987	Increase 1971-87 %
Occupational therapists	3359	9306	177.0
Dietitians	930	2584	177.8
Orthoptists	620	966	155.8
Medical laboratory technicians	7918	20134	154.3
Radiographers	8171	15160	85.5
Physiotherapists	10933	19780	80.9
Chiropodists	4657	6142	31.9
Total	36588	74072	102.4

members are registered by the CPSM, with the exception of the much smaller group of dietitians (Table 2) – it has clearly not been great enough to permit every established post to be filled.

Since 1963, when the CPSM's registers first started, a total of some 16,200 individuals have registered as occupational therapists, while 7,000 have left the register. Deaths, retirements, migration and other compelling reasons will have accounted for the majority of those who have left. Nevertheless, given the number of newly qualified occupational therapists joining the register each year, who must be many more than those leaving for such reasons, it is clear that there must be a pool of qualified professionals of working age in the UK who are not registering because they are not working – at least not in occupational therapy posts.

It is a common experience in professions composed predominantly of women, like occupational therapy, that young, newly qualified individuals will leave employment, at least temporarily, when they start to bear and rear children. The statutory provision of paid maternity leave, sometimes topped up by additional employer-based financial and other arrangements, may have marginally increased the number of women for whom absence is minimal. But there is a general consensus among labour economists and equal opportunity advocates that the financial incentives associated with work in predominantly female occupations are insufficient to stem an outflow of those in their late twenties and early thirties, which tends to become permanent rather than temporary. This is particularly so for professions in the public sector where employers are more constrained than those in private sector enterprises in their ability to give incentives for women to return to work.

Our own survey threw some light on the reasons why

occupational therapists left posts during the 12-month period to 31 March 1988. During that time 1217 NHS staff left their posts (see Appendix B, Table 9). Most of them, however, remained in the profession: 915 merely changed their posts within the NHS (558 were promoted, 319 moved horizontally to other posts in the same grade, and 38 were demoted on moving): 113 went to local authority employment, and 74 went abroad, 28 of the latter being foreign or Commonwealth nationals returning to their own country.

The survey data, however, indicated that 115 NHS staff left the profession, and this represented as much as 4% of all the established posts included in the survey. To this must be added 98 individuals leaving the profession from the 82 responding local authorities surveyed. Predictably, a large number, especially of the qualified, left to have babies and another 75, 39 of them qualified, left for domestic reasons. Ill-health and retirement together took very few of the qualified but substantial numbers of helpers and technical instructors (Table 3). What is worrying for the profession, however, is the relatively large numbers of both qualified OTs and other staff leaving for another career altogether. Nevertheless it should be appreciated that the categories of reasons given in the questionnaires were not entirely satisfactory, and

Table 3. Reasons for leaving NHS OT posts

Reasons given	Qualified		Unqualified		Total	
	N	%	N	%	N	%
Another career	30	12	101	33	131	24
Maternity	85	34	17	6	102	19
Domestic	39	16	36	12	75	14
Retirement	15	6	54	18	69	13
Ill-health	8	3	24	8	32	6
All other reasons + unknown	70	28	70	23	140	25
Total	247	99	302	99	549	100

the results given in Table 3 should not be assumed to be an entirely accurate reflection of the true situation.

The survey data also showed the provenance of those who came into NHS and LASS posts in the 12 months before 31 March 1988. About 8% of all established NHS posts were filled by new recruits, most of them entering the Basic grade category. Not surprisingly, most of the intake to Senior posts was from the Basic grade, but 92 of them re-entered the NHS after a 'break' – presumably occasioned for domestic, including maternity, reasons. In LASS employment the largest number of those who joined posts in the year re-entered after a 'break'. It was something of a surprise to find that in only 22 of the posts filled in LASS departments during the year were the entrants direct from NHS posts, compared with 79 NHS posts filled by entrants from the LASS departments.

We found, during our visits to different departments, that many departmental heads were concerned at what they considered to be unacceptably high wastage rates among their staff, although some thought the rates were dropping. In our view, however, the departmental heads lacked comparisons with other professions against which their own department's performance could be measured. Indeed they usually failed to take into account some of the factors influencing the work decisions of young, professionally qualified women in an expanding occupation. It is to such considerations that attention is now turned.

The dynamics of expanding professions

There is a considerable literature on manpower analysis which demonstrates how institutions, firms and professions are vulnerable when they go through periods of rapid, sustained growth, such as that being experienced by the OT profession. When expansion begins, the age-profile immediately changes – the average age falling as the number of recruits increases. As more senior posts are created to manage the growing system, newcomers have excellent promotion prospects – much better than the innate structure of the system really justifies. An early report (1981) by a working party of occupational therapists in the SE Thames region vividly illustrates this. At the time 46% of Basic grade occupational therapists remained in post for less than a year, either because they had been promoted or because they had left the job. As the newly promoted managers in such circumstances tend to be young, they are likely to remain in the system longer, so that the promotion prospects of following cohorts of recruits begin to diminish, though this tendency may not be apparent for some time, since it is masked by the continuing creation of additional senior posts as long as expansion continues. If expansion slows down or stops, promotion rates are bound to fall, promotion itself becoming a question of waiting for dead men's shoes. Eventually those managers who benefited by rapid promotion in the early stages of expansion begin to retire and a second round of improved promotion prospects begins. In short, rapid expansion inevitably introduces long-lasting conditions of boom and slump in promotion prospects and eventually for new recruits. In the second phase younger members can become frustrated when they see that their predecessors have advanced further and faster than they are likely to, and their frustration may induce higher rates of leaving. We believe that the profession of occupational therapy has been experiencing such changes, which account for much of the malaise felt among its members.

When the profession is composed largely of women, other factors influence their working patterns besides promotion prospects. The rate of women's return to work after raising a family varies from profession to profession, depending on the location and availability of appropriate work. If such work is available near home they are more able to return when their children are comparatively young. If not, they are faced with the problem of having to travel longish distances and will be less able to accept work. They may therefore be lost to their original profession because they will choose to take up other work if the opportunity arises to get back to work sooner. It is an observed fact that the longer a woman remains out of her original profession the less likely she is to return to work in it. We lack information on the career histories of qualified OTs no longer in NHS or LASS posts; but we believe that the concentration of posts in the hospital sector of the NHS may have made it more difficult for some of those who have left for domestic reasons in early or mid-career to return to occupational therapy than it has been in school-teaching and nursing, where there is a more widespread geographical distribution of appropriate professional work.

Evidence to support this contention came from a small survey carried out in 1987 in the Leicestershire Health Authority by Maxine Blumfield and Clare Greensmith, which was made available to us. They reported that in the NHS sector the occupational therapists were predominantly young – in the age group 21-25 – and that only 57% were married. In LASS the age distribution was much more even across all age groups, and 81% were married. It can be inferred from this that OTs can more readily find work near their homes with LASS departments than in the NHS. Furthermore 40% of occupational therapists working in the NHS told the investigators that they had considered leaving, as against only 21% of those working in LASS departments.

Oral and written evidence from various regions appears to support such findings.

We also obtained unquantifiable evidence about another feature of the manpower position which is likely to apply to small professional groups such as occupational therapy, as opposed for example to large ones such as medicine or nursing. The young, newly appointed OT is likely to find herself working in some isolation from her fellow professionals. Very early in her career she has to take responsibility for decision-making affecting the welfare of her clients, and she may be in charge of helpers who are her superiors in age and working experience. She may lack the supervision, care and support she needs. This is another factor leading to insecurity and frustration which, in turn, lead to higher staff wastage. When an occupational therapist who does stay through this initial period leaves to have a family, her early experiences may condition her attitude to returning to work. It is a common experience among professional women that, when practice and technology are changing quickly – as they are in occupational therapy – they worry about being out-of-date if and when they return.

Given these kinds of circumstance, we believe that it is worth emphasising the profession's need to provide support and encouragement to young Basic grade OTs at the start of their careers and to promote carefully constructed reinduction training for those who return after a break.

Forecasts of the number of occupational therapists needed to meet future demand

It was not clear to us how the College arrived at its estimate of the need for a 73% expansion in the number of qualified occupational therapists. So we tried to make our own forecast by applying the norms published by the

College in two documents – one for the NHS and the other for the LASS.[3] It was not easy to interpret or use either document, so that one of our recommendations is that they should be revised and updated and the norms for both employing authorities coordinated, so that overall needs for a given population can be derived from them.

Applying the 1980 norms to the NHS specialty bed numbers for England as in 1985[4] suggests that the required ratio of *qualified* occupational therapists in the NHS per 1000 current population should be at least 0.19, rather than the achieved 0.10 found in our survey. If the 1984 estimate for residential and day care units provided by LASS departments is increased to allow for sickness and leave cover, it gives a figure of 0.017 *qualified* per 1000. If it is assumed that half the OT staff in LASS are qualified, this ratio corresponds to that found in our survey. Adding the NHS and LASS estimates together gives a recommended ratio of 0.21 *qualified* OTs per 1000 population, which contrasts sharply with the present ratio of filled posts of 0.12.

In our view, however, even this ratio is too low to enable the profession to meet its obligations to potential patients and clients. A 3.5% increase in total population is expected by the year 2001, including a projected increase of 14% in the elderly (75 and over). A projection of the increase in disability due to these demographic changes suggests a further increase of at least 10% in the ratio. This does not take into account the increased requirement for qualified occupational therapists in response to the expected shortening of hospital stays and

[3] 'Recommended minimum standards for occupational therapy staff patient ratios', COT 1980; and 'Community occupational therapy. Future needs and numbers', COT 1984.
[4] Health and Personal Social Services Statistics, 1987.

increasing emphasis on community care. These factors, in our view, call for yet another 10% on the estimated ratio. The resultant figure reached by us is therefore 0.25 qualified occupational therapists per 1000 population, more than twice the current ratio based on filled posts.

Bearing in mind the projected increase in the population, this would predicate a need for not far short of 15,000 qualified occupational therapists in posts in the UK by the end of the century to serve a population of about 59 million. Roughly 12,500 of them would be required for England, 1,300 for Scotland, 750 for Wales and 450 for Northern Ireland. The College's estimate of the need for a 73% expansion is, in our view, too low. Our own estimate is for an 80% expansion.[5]

Recruitment in the future

Hitherto the profession has been remarkably successful in recruiting to its training schools teenagers with the capacity to acquire the basic knowledge and skills required to work as occupational therapists. The number starting to train in 1979 was 767, and by 1988 it had increased to 891, plus a further 62 mainly unqualified helpers, on in-service courses. Encouragingly, the last few years have also seen a growing number of mature students aged 25 or more. In 1988 22.3% of the intake to the schools were so classed.

Drop-out rates during training have been variable between schools, and remain so. Catherine Paterson, however, records a substantial fall in national annual drop-out rates during the 1980s, estimating the 1983

[5] Neither COT document specifically suggests the ideal ratio of qualified to unqualified staff, although the LASS document included a table implying a one-to-one ratio. A later chapter deals with various aspects of the relation of qualified to unqualified staff.

rate at about 15% compared with rates between 20% and 29% in the early 1970s.[6] Such a rate is much greater than in medicine, but smaller than for state-registered nursing.

A surprising finding of our own survey is the small number of newly qualified recruits who take up posts in the NHS and LASS compared with the numbers who graduate. For example, only some 440 took up posts in the 12 months to 31 March 1988, although 690 had graduated from the schools in 1987. This discrepancy seems large and needs further investigation. The profession cannot expand at the rate needed if so many of its graduates fail to take up work on qualification.

Finally, we do not need to remind representatives of the profession that it is likely to be much more difficult in the 1990s to maintain the rate of recruitment to the profession from school leavers achieved during the 1980s, let alone *increase* it to meet norms of the order recommended. The numbers in the 16-19 age group – those set to start work or training for work – will fall by over a quarter between 1989 and 1994. The shortage of recruits is already being felt in nursing and school-teaching, both much larger professions than occupational therapy. As in school-teaching they recruit mainly among women and from women who probably have much the same work motivations and ambitions, and educational standards, as occupational therapists. The conclusion is that the OT profession must look forward to a continuing period of increased competition for the smaller number of potential recruits.

Some other similarly placed professions have decided to try to improve their attraction to teenagers of the

[6] C.F. Paterson, 'Annual survey of occupational therapy students: reasons for drop-out', *British Journal of Occupational Therapy*, March 1988.

intellectual calibre needed by making the basic professional qualification a degree rather than a diploma. There are those in the College who believe that it is necessary for the profession to take a similar course, if only not to be excluded from the pool of potential talent. It is also argued that the present diploma is of at least the intellectual standard required for an ordinary degree in many subjects. Against this, it is claimed that many potentially good occupational therapists come from those whose talents are practical rather than academic. Making it obligatory for all entrants to reach degree standard would, it is thought, reduce the pool of potentially good recruits to the profession.

Given the competition from different professions for the hearts and minds, not only of a diminishing number of school leavers but also of a substantial pool of mature women who have completed their families and/or wish to change their life course, it is essential for the future of occupational therapy that a firm decision be taken in the near future on the direction the profession should take. We considered the matter at some length, recognising the advantages and disadvantages of the various choices before the College. This is further discussed in Chapter 4 and our recommendation is given in Chapter 7.

3

Role, Function and Organisation

In Chapter 1, a brief description was given of the demographic factors and advances in medicine which together led earlier in this century to the establishment of occupational therapy as an integral component of the country's health and welfare service provision. It was followed in Chapter 2 by an account of the phenomenal growth which has taken place in the last two decades in the numbers of OTs employed in the National Health Service and, to a lesser extent, in the Local Authority Social Services. Chapter 2 also showed how occupational therapists were currently deployed in various hospital-based specialties and the Community services of the NHS as well as in Local Authority Social Services departments. It concluded that, despite the expansion in the numbers of qualified occupational therapists, their unqualified helpers and their technical instructors, the demand for individuals with the basic requisite knowledge and skills was not being currently met in most parts of the country in any of the branches of the health and social services which needed them. It was further concluded that, if anything, potential demand would be even greater if it were not artificially suppressed by the continuing failure to supply the numbers required, particularly in the Basic grade of the profession.

43

We are mindful that we are reporting at a time when the practices and procedures of all professional groups and public sector enterprises are being subjected to intense scrutiny. Given the determination of central government to evaluate every aspect of its great national commitment – the NHS – and of the personal social services sector for which local government is at present responsible, occupational therapy cannot be exempted from this overall review and the possible strategic redeployment of its forces, even if members of the profession were to wish it otherwise. We believe that our conclusions, reached after a consideration of possible options open to the profession, may help the College of Occupational Therapists and its members to respond with greater confidence to the challenge which this degree of Government re-thinking has set them.

In this chapter, therefore, we consider:

(1) Whether the activities undertaken by occupational therapists and their helpers are essential components of modern health care, or whether, in straitened economic circumstances, they could be dispensed with altogether or in part without harming individuals.

(2) Whether any of the activities currently undertaken by occupational therapists could be adequately performed by less highly qualified professional workers.

(3) Whether there is a case for a generic rehabilitation worker in place of the various professions whose work may possibly overlap with that of the occupational therapist.

(4) Whether the greater concentration of occupational therapists in the hospital-based specialties, as opposed to the community services of the NHS and local government, can be justified, or whether the time has come for an organisational re-alignment of the profession towards the community.

3. Role, Function and Organisation

In the next chapter, we report on the present recruitment and training of occupational therapists, and give our recommendations for the changes in them which we consider should flow from the conclusions reached in this chapter.

Is occupational therapy really necessary?

While not subscribing to the maxim that every profession is inevitably a conspiracy against the laity, we recognise that all professions, in seeking to maintain public confidence in their performance in the particular field of activity in which they claim exclusive competence, may have a vested interest in exaggerating the benefits to be derived from their services. They may also claim that such services cannot be satisfactorily or safely undertaken by those who have not, after certain preliminary educational credentials, successfully accomplished training of the intensity and quality which their members have undergone.

In considering how far occupational therapy, as it has evolved in its relatively short lifetime, can be said to be of unquestionable benefit to those who have received it, we appreciated that we could not draw on the 'hard' data which would wholly satisfy the sceptic, the scientist or the cost-conscious health service manager. In the first place there were no available accounts of experiments in which patients with comparable rehabilitation needs were randomly allocated to treatment either by teams containing occupational therapists or by those without them. In the second place, we could not ourselves commission opinion surveys among doctors or social workers who had referred patients for occupational therapy, let alone among representative samples of the patients who had received it.

We believe that the virtual absence of experimental research designed to evaluate the effectiveness of occupational therapy practices and procedures, as well as of surveys designed to test patient response to OT services, is a weakness which leaves the profession unnecessarily vulnerable to challenge and which, therefore, it should take energetic steps to remedy. It is, of course, a weakness shared with other health professions, and is understandable, given the absence of research emphasis in basic training and the limited opportunities offered to pursue research in most practice positions. In the present climate affecting decision-making in health and social services, those professions which seek successfully to evaluate their practices are likely to gain the advantage over those which do not.

We did, however, obtain a considerable volume of evidence during the course of our work which served to convince us that there is a real need for occupational therapy and a widespread appreciation of the work undertaken by occupational therapists and their helpers. As might be expected, many members of the profession itself who responded to the request for information on their activities laid claim to achievements which were short of perfection only because of pressure of work or the failure of other professional groups to screen appropriate clients. What was impressive, however, was the response from bodies representing other health professions, in particular those concerned with rehabilitation. Almost universally these bodies indicated that their members regarded the work of occupational therapists as indispensable and high praise was often given to its quality. These favourable opinions were reinforced by the more anecdotal accounts which we obtained informally when we questioned doctors, nurses and social workers, as well as recipients of service, during our visits to health service establishments.

As a result, any doubts that any of us – all of us independent of the profession, it should be remembered – may have had at the outset about the value of work which could be best undertaken by individuals with the specific and unique combination of knowledge and skills acquired in occupational therapy training (see Chapter 1) were dispelled at the finish. In our view, for many, if not most of those who have experienced acute illness or trauma serious enough to require hospital treatment, as well as for many of those with chronic disabilities and handicaps, whether predominantly physical or mental, living in their own homes or in residential institutions, an occupational therapist is the health professional best equipped to comprehend and meet their needs.

Can occupational therapy tasks be undertaken by less highly trained personnel?

Given the shortfall in the number of occupational therapists to which we have drawn attention, it is clear that at present work which optimally should be done by fully qualified professional workers is, in many instances, performed by helpers who lack the systematic training of the occupational therapist. Moreover some of the evidence we received suggested that health service managers as well as doctors and nurses were sometimes unaware that patients referred for occupational therapy might be dealt with by unqualified and possibly unsupervised staff. This ignorance is combined with the continued demeaning stereotype of occupational therapy as a limited activity of do-gooders, rather than as the product of a sophisticated diagnosis of life needs by highly trained professionals. The result of the combination of shortages of fully qualified occupational therapists and negative stereotypes of the profession is to support those who, for whatever reason, are prone to give comparatively low priority to the proper staffing of occupational therapy departments.

In our view one of the most persuasive arguments for the need for a full complement of trained occupational therapists in the hospital specialties where there is a demand for occupational therapy services, as well as in the community services, is the widespread desire among untrained helpers themselves for further training (see Chapter 5). In short those who are forced, faute de mieux, to undertake assessments and procedures for which they are not trained recognise their own inadequacy and seek to remedy it.

At the same time we recognise that excessive workloads placed on under-staffed departments can distort perspectives, and it would be surprising if occupational therapists were not sometimes undertaking work which could equally well be done by helpers or by clerical staff. This can happen when a department is reluctant to refuse referrals made to it despite its patent inability to provide a proper service. It is a problem which is most likely to arise when the staff in charge are junior, inexperienced and perhaps too anxious to please. Paradoxically it can cause unproductive stress and ultimately a reluctance to remain in or rejoin the profession after a break for family-building. We know that the College is aware of this problem. Here we simply wish to stress our own view, expressed elsewhere, that continuing support and guidance for its neophytes is essential if the profession is to weather the hazards facing occupational groups which are both expanding and composed largely of women. The problem is likely to become more, not less, difficult to resolve in the next decade given the reduced size of the pool of late teenagers from which occupational therapy, in common with other professions, must draw most of its recruits.

What is required is a rigorous review of procedures and conventions, which may have become entrenched in a time warp, in order to eliminate wasteful and unproductive activities and ensure the best use of limited personnel resources.

Should there be a generalist rehabilitation professional worker to replace the present separate remedial professions?

We came to the conclusion that the answer to the question posed in this sub-heading must be in the negative, at least for the foreseeable future, although we did not rule out the need to keep the question – certainly not a purely rhetorical one – under review. Some of us indeed thought that the matter should be given detailed consideration immediately.

The physiotherapists have been joined recently by the remedial gymnasts – admittedly a small group numerically – who are engaged in rehabilitation, so that a process of unification can be said to have begun. Viewed from the outside, the case for ending the primary distinction between the physiotherapists and the occupational therapists, the two major professions involved in rehabilitation, is a strong one.

First, there is undoubtedly some overlap in the functions of the two professions, especially in the rehabilitation of patients suffering from the effects of somatic illnesses, such as osteoarthritis, and of trauma. Existing demarcation divisions of task can appear to the outsider as arbitrary rather than functional from the viewpoint of the recipients, who usually want to minimise the number of individuals in the caring professions with whom they have to deal.

Second, there has been some narrowing of the differences in the basic training of the two professions. Physiotherapists still concentrate to a much greater extent than occupational therapists on the anatomy and physiology of the human body and on physical procedures required to restore damaged function; but their basic courses lay increasing emphasis on the social and psychological factors influencing response to their work and on the suitability of employment and of leisure occupations for patients in the long, as well as the short, term.

Third, it can be argued that the existence of two professions in the same health-care field both confuses other health professions and managers and presents them – not always falsely – as competing with each other for scarce resources instead of combining to promote rehabilitation generally. Twenty years ago the ending of historical divisions in the social work field and the creation of a unified profession resulted in an improvement in its overall standing and authority in both community and hospital-based services. A single occupational group, albeit with post-qualification specialisation as in medicine, might serve to enhance the status of rehabilitation work as a whole. Even after unification, the profession would still be minuscule compared with the other professional groups which absorb most women – teaching, nursing and social work.

Fourth, given the current reduction in the numbers entering further education and the world of work, it would make sense for two occupations with comparable objectives and overlapping functions to combine resources in order better to compete – as compete they must – with other potential professions for the hearts and minds of those capable of performing well in these vital caring tasks.

3. Role, Function and Organisation

Those who advocate the creation of a unified rehabilitation profession do not deny the need for some specialisation in practice. It may be appropriate for some individuals to concentrate on the physical aspects of restoring function, while others would necessarily work on the socio-psychological aspects of longer-term life adjustment. A common basic training – of say 18 months – might give way later to 18 months of more specialised training designed to steer individuals into one or other of these fields. Post-registration supervised and evaluated experience would endorse the choice of specialisation, which might further differentiate the area of specialisation – for example, into the growing field of work with mentally handicapped patients, as compared with those of psychiatric or elderly patients and of adolescent and early adult traumatised patients.

There are several cogent arguments, however, some of substance and some of sentiment, against amalgamation of the two branches of therapists. Each branch has an established network of training institutions, whose work would be seriously disrupted if the two professions were to merge. There is already enough turmoil in the public sector health and welfare services not to court more by imposing new structures which are not strictly essential and not desired by those involved. Given too that post-qualification specialisation – replicating to a large extent the present division of tasks between occupational and physiotherapists – would continue to be required, the benefit to be derived in efficiency from merging is unlikely to be great, at least in the short run. Finally, each profession, although comparatively young, has acquired its own distinct traditions and characteristics, and most members – at any rate of the numerically smaller profession, occupational therapy – would feel an acute sense of loss if their special identity were to be lost in the larger whole.

Should occupational therapy redeploy its forces from the hospital to the community?

An even more important consideration for the future of the profession, in our opinion, is how far its members should continue to be employed predominantly in the hospital sector of the NHS.

There are good historical reasons, which we need not rehearse here, why occupational therapy as a specialised professional health service originated and until recently thrived in the hospital sector. However, current and future demographic changes and the development of medical technology now call for a substantial transfer of resources from the hospital to the community.

In earlier chapters attention was drawn to the effect of an ageing population suffering more commonly from chronic disabling conditions than acute infections, on the character of the health enterprise generally and on the demand for occupational therapy services in particular. Here it is necessary to emphasise the actual and projected impact of developments in medical, surgical and psychiatric technology and procedures on the future deployment of health personnel, including occupational therapists, as between hospital and community.

Changes in medical and surgical practice have resulted in an increasingly fast through-put in the acute hospital sector, resulting in shortened lengths of stay for nearly all patients. Combined with increasing emphasis on cost containment, early discharge already means that more and more of the process of patient recovery from medical and surgical interventions, including convalesence and rehabilitation, now takes place outside the hospital. The incentives for hospitals to maximise the use of their expensive facilities are likely to increase still further and to lead to even greater pressures on them to discharge patients who, not so long ago, would have expected to spend days or weeks undergoing rehabilitative diagnosis and therapy while still occupying a hospital bed.

These changes in the acute hospital specialties dealing with somatic illness and injury have been paralleled by substantial changes in the treatment of psychiatric patients. In the last decade many large psychiatric hospitals – mostly built in the Victorian era – have greatly reduced their number of beds. First, admission for a psychiatric condition is now mainly to a ward in a district general hospital where the objective is rapid assessment and discharge for care in the community – in a hostel or at home. Where possible, patients with long-term psychotic complaints, as well as those with considerable mental handicaps, are now seen as ideally located in their own family home or in a hostel rather than in a hospital.

If occupational therapy is to play the part in patient care, which we believe it can and should, the profession must not ignore the logic of these trends. In our view that logic calls for a considerable shift in the location of the profession's members. Patients who can be helped by occupational therapy will, for the most part, be out there, in their own homes, in residential institutions or in hostels. The preponderance of occupational therapists in the hospital sector (80%) must be replaced by a preponderance in the community care sector (20%). The process has already begun but, in the coming decade, the pace must be accelerated.

To say this is not to suggest that the hospitals should be evacuated wholesale by the profession. There will still be a need for hospitals – particularly in mental handicap and geriatrics – where patients may stay for considerable lengths of time, and they will undoubtedly require the services of the occupational therapists and their helpers.

There should also be some staff working with doctors and nurses in the acute hospital specialties to identify individual needs for occupational therapy and to give advice and make the necessary referrals to community-based services.

The Commission members recognise that the prescription for such a substantial redeployment may not be palatable to every member of the profession. It will mean, for some, leaving the familiar, supportive and prestigious location of the hospital. Moreover, at the time of writing (June 1989), the Government's intentions for the future shape of the community care services and responsibility for their management are still not clear. The Griffiths Report (*Community Care: Agenda for Action, 1987*), made certain recommendations, notably that local government should be responsible for overseeing the provision of all community care facilities, including those in the private and voluntary sectors, which were generally welcomed by those already engaged in community care.

Assuming, however, as we have been compelled to do, that the Griffiths proposals, or something very close to them, will become Government policy, a redeployment of OT forces to the community services will involve the profession in many contingent moves. In the circumstances it is impossible to be specific, but these moves will probably include:

(1) Shifts in the practice locations to which occupational therapy students are sent during their training.

(2) Negotiations with Directors of Social Services and others to ensure the suitable positioning of occupational therapists in social service districts and the expansion of day and other centres for patient assessment and treatment.

(3) Consideration of the expansion of career posts for

qualified occupational therapists in local government, and the opportunity to occupy general management posts at all levels.

(4) Clarification of the relationships and levels of responsibility enjoyed by qualified occupational therapists and the many different kinds of rehabilitation-oriented workers at present employed in local government.

(5) Possible placements of occupational therapists and/or helpers in large group general practice units.

It cannot be pretended that the proposal the Commission is making for community redeployment is likely to be easy or problem-free. We should warn, for example, against the mistake we believe was committed by the social work profession when the social services departments of local authorities were established in 1971. This was to claim too much for its own capacity to meet needs. Such a danger awaits occupational therapy too, where there is such a huge, unmet demand for aids and appliances to make life easier for elderly and handicapped people, and where expectations can all too easily be raised.

In 1971 it was not envisaged that occupational therapists would play a major role in the newly formed social services departments, and members of the sister profession of social work, whose training and skills overlap to some extent that of occupational therapists, have naturally tended to entrench themselves in the departments and to react defensively to suggestions that other professionals may be as well-suited as they are to contribute to their management and development. The Commission does not wish to see an internecine struggle for power between two professions, who share not only many of the same problems but also the same overall objectives for human welfare. It believes that both are mature enough to recognise that their own good lies in close collaboration in the overriding interest of their patients and clients.

To summarise, then, the conclusions of this chapter. They are, first, that occupational therapy is needed as an integral part of health and social service provision; second, that although there is room for a devolution of some of the work at present performed by trained occupational therapists to their helpers and clerical staff, there will be a continuing and expanding need for fully professional occupational therapists; third, that further consideration should be given, in the long-term if not in the immediate future, to the creation of a united profession of rehabilitation therapists, permitting post-qualification specialisation; and fourth, that in the next decade and increasingly into the twenty-first century occupational therapy should be largely relocated in the community care services.

4

Recruitment, Preparation and Qualification

In previous chapters, we indicated that we saw the need for even greater numbers of occupational therapists to perform the functions in the health and social services for which their present education in knowledge and training in skills equips them. At the same time we drew attention to the diminished pool of teenagers which can be expected in the next decade and from which the major part of their recruits must be drawn.

In this chapter, we consider the problems which face the profession as a result of the need to expand numbers at a time when expansion is likely to become more difficult. The issues of recruitment, preparation and qualification are all bound up with one another; but here it is proposed to spend more time on the relationship between recruitment and qualification, and less on preparation. This is because we believe that, by and large, the training colleges have got their educational packages about right, as regards both the knowledge content of their courses and the acquisition of skills in the basic training period. Moreover we believe that, even if the present diploma were to be replaced eventually by a degree as the basic professional qualification – an issue considered later in this chapter – there will be little need to undertake fundamental restructuring of existing courses. Naturally greater modification may be required in basic courses if the profession decides, in the long run, to join forces with physiotherapists to form a single rehabilitation profession.

Recruitment

Since occupational therapy is a small profession, it follows that school leavers contemplating a career in a caring profession are much less likely to have met an occupational therapist than say a nurse or a social worker, let alone have been helped by one. In 1987 there were roughly 2,000 applicants to the 16 UK schools: 844 of them were ultimately admitted. It is not known exactly how many of the unsuccessful applicants were rejected because they lacked either the minimum academic entrance requirements or the personal characteristics which the college selectors felt those intent on joining the profession should possess. Some suitable applicants indeed may have withdrawn after being offered a place. Whatever the truth of the matter, it is clear that the training schools, at present, have to select from a very small number of applicants.

If, as we expect, the profession recruits an increasing proportion of the diminishing pool of candidates interested in a career in a caring profession, it should certainly review its current methods of publicising its needs to schools career officers and others. It must ensure that information about career possibilities and training places is readily available throughout the country. A Central Admissions System, run by the College of Occupational Therapists, is of crucial significance.

Entrance requirements

At this point, it should be asked whether it would be easier to recruit to the profession if the academic entrance qualifications demanded by the schools were to be reduced. At present these normally require applicants to have five or six GCEs (or GCSEs), at least two of which should be at 'A' level. Some schools specify subjects, most calling for an 'O' level in English language and in mathematics or a science subject. These, be it noted, are no less than the *minimum* requirements set by many universities and polytechnics for students proposing to study for a degree, although, at present, most faculties insist that entrants achieve high grades in what they regard as relevant subjects.

In our view it would not be sensible for the profession to reduce its entrance requirements, at least for school leavers, in the hope that by so doing they could attract more recruits. In the first place the successful completion of training does require at least the intellectual capacity and prior educational attainment represented by the present entry requirements. If school leavers do not possess them, it is likely to indicate either that they lack the capacity and/or persistence required to profit by the OT courses, or (for example, if they have left school at the earliest possible moment) that they have not yet reached a firm decision about a future career. In either case they are unlikely to prove satisfied or satisfactory recruits to the profession.

We support the policy of suspending minimum entry requirements for mature applicants, in order to treat each one on its merits. Given demographic trends, more and more of the profession's recruits will come from mature women who have completed their family-building, during which period they have acquired the kind of experience, wisdom and skills which are needed in the caring professions. Some will have been early school-leavers whose capacity for serious and persistent study had not then been tested. Many will have discovered a vocation by working as an unqualified helper or assistant in a caring profession. In recommending that the profession do their utmost to encourage recruitment of this kind, we are simply underlining a move which has already started and which we believe should be pursued even more vigorously. Chapter 5 contains our recommendations concerning in-service courses for top-grade helpers.

It is also important for the profession to attract to its ranks, as to some extent it already has, as many graduates as it can from the range of academic disciplines which have something to offer occupational therapy. Indeed it can be argued that few, if any, academic disciplines have no relevance to the practice of occupational therapy. It can benefit from the knowledge and critical insights which those who have studied the natural sciences, the arts, philosophy, psychology and the social sciences can bring to it. If such recruitment is to take place on any scale, it is essential to provide accelerated qualification courses, and to publicise the attractions of the profession among university and polytechnic careers advisers.

Preparation: the basic course

Whether or not a unified generic rehabilitation profession emerges in the future, one question that must be asked is whether it is appropriate to train all recruits to be equipotent in the physical and psychiatric fields. In our view it is certainly necessary that all occupational therapists, in the first part of their basic course, should have a general grounding in the knowledge and skills required for work with both physically disabled and mentally disordered patients. This core, which should last for the first 18 months to two years of the three year basic course, would comprise general theory as well as one practice placement in a situation dealing predominantly with the rehabilitation of those with physical disabilities and another in a situation where the problems are primarily mental. There is a powerful argument for a degree of specialisation in one or other of these fields during the remaining months of the basic course before qualification, involving a more specialised theoretical course in one or other field, together with further appropriate placements.

Preparation: post-qualification supervision

We also think that the claims of occupational therapists to undisputed professional status would be enhanced if the registering body were to withhold full registration from diploma or degree holders until after the completion of at least one year's post-qualification supervised work. Once this pre-registration period had been completed to the satisfaction of a qualified practitioner, full registration would be confirmed. Elsewhere we have indicated that some of the profession's current difficulties appear to arise because unblooded recruits have often to work in unsupervised posts and undertake daunting responsibilities. Continuing shortages affecting basic grade positions may make this recommendation difficult to implement in the short term; but it is important that the profession should signal its intent to move in this direction.

Preparation: the teachers

Later in this chapter we suggest that the 'monocultural' institutions (to use the latest jargon), in which occupational therapy training has taken place historically, should join with universities and/or polytechnics in order, among other things, to exploit their teaching and research potential as well as to enhance the image of the profession as one of the occupations whose preparation takes place in the country's mainstream higher educational establishments.

Here it is important to emphasise another concern. In our visits to various occupational therapy training schools and practice settings we found some dissatisfaction with the equivocal position of those in practice settings who were acting as supervisors for students during their placements. Equally some disquiet was expressed about teachers in the colleges, who may have had previous formal experience of professional working, but who could easily get out of date and lose touch with recent developments in practice settings.

To safeguard against twin dangers of this kind, we felt that the profession should encourage regular secondment of teachers to practice situations and vice versa. Closer collaboration between those responsible for the profession's neophytes in both their initial training and subsequent work settings can only benefit the profession as a whole.

The qualification: diploma or degree?

We are convinced that the academic level attained by those who gain the Diploma in Occupational Therapy – the profession's basic qualification – is at least as high as that achieved by students taking an ordinary degree in

English or Scottish universities and polytechnics. The question we felt compelled to ask, therefore, was whether the time had not come for the profession to enter formally into negotiations with the CNAA and/or individual universities to transform the present diploma courses into degree courses.

There are arguments for and against such a proposal. One of the first considerations must be its likely effect on recruitment, and this is difficult to forecast. Some of those at present attracted to the profession may be essentially practical, pragmatic individuals who only seek a licence to practise rather than an academic qualification. They may be put off by the degree. In particular a degree requirement may deter some of the mature women who are now attracted to the profession.

On the other hand, some of those who would make excellent occupational therapists may choose to enter other professions which either require a degree as an entry qualification or discriminate more positively in favour of degree entrants than does occupational therapy. After all, it is only human to resent being the recipient of a qualification which has a lower status than that awarded to others who have expended no more time and effort in attaining it.

The issue the profession has to face is not new. However, the recent decision of the Chartered Society of Physiotherapists to transform their profession into an 'all-graduate' one lends urgency to the debate. We believe that if the College of Occupational Therapists does not promptly take at least the initial steps to achieve the same end in the long run, it will be in danger of being left behind in the competition for a fair share of the kind of recruits from among school leavers for which it is looking. It will also prove more difficult to attract university and polytechnic graduates from a variety of disciplines into its ranks. Such recruits are needed above all to strengthen the research-based justification for the profession's practices and procedures which, at present, is sorely lacking.

In recommending that the profession take steps to achieve degree status for its basic qualification, we wish to make clear that we are not thinking of an honours degree. A general or ordinary degree is the attainment level for qualified people in the professions supplementary to medicine in all countries with an equivalent level of health service provision, and we consider that it should be so in this country as well. Moreover, in the light of developments now taking place in the higher education sector, the conferment of graduate status on qualified occupational therapists would also make them more easily eligible for admission to higher and research degrees.

We see a further advantage accruing to the profession from a move to graduate status. While we have been impressed with the high educational and training standards attained by the schools of occupational therapy which we visited, and welcome in particular the innovatory degree courses already established in three schools and projected for the remaining two Scottish schools in the immediate future, we believe that the profession has much to gain from the close collaboration of its educational establishments with the multi-disciplinary, multi-faculty institutions of the higher education sector as a whole. Isolated colleges can turn in on themselves to the detriment of staff and students. For both the loss is likely to be academic – in the sense of restricted sources of intellectual stimulation – and social. Now that the polytechnic sector has gained a considerable degree of independence from local authority bureaucracy, it is almost everywhere exploring new ways of developing its educational contribution, particularly for the many professional groups who provide health and social services for the country. It is essential that occupational therapy should be well represented in the negotiations now taking place. The elitism of the university sector too, which once served to exclude all but a handful of learned professions and to denigrate occupations requiring the acquisition of human relations and practical skills, is for various reasons more and more a thing of the past. Opportunities exist for professions whose members are as highly regarded and as much in demand as that of occupational therapy to take their rightful place in the institutions of higher education.

To summarise, we consider that the profession should not vary – either by increasing or by lowering – the entry requirements for its school-leaving age recruits. We urge the College of Occupational Therapists to see that the attractions of the profession are better known in schools and in universities and colleges. We hope, however, that even more encouragement will be given to mature women to join the profession. In this instance we suggest the waiving, where necessary, of the academic achievements required of school leavers.

We believe that the present curricula and practical training offered in schools of occupational therapy are about right, and that they are of general degree standard. In our view future recruitment will be easier and justice will be done if the present diploma is recognised by degree awarding bodies as the equivalent of an ordinary degree. We think further that the professional training institutions should develop closer association with universities and polytechnics in order to give staff and students fuller use of their multi-disciplinary, multi-faculty facilities, especially in order to promote cooperation with other health professional groups.

5

Helpers and Technical Instructors

The primary objective of our briefing was to advise the profession on the best course it should be taking to meet the community's needs for occupational therapy into the twenty-first century and the interests of the qualified members of the profession. Those issues were dealt with in the first two chapters, and are taken up again in Chapter 6 where we consider the negotiating arrangements for determining salaries and conditions of work.

The activities which constitute the work of occupational therapy departments in the NHS, however, or of comparable sections going under a variety of names in LASS departments, are not carried out solely by qualified occupational therapists. For every 100 qualified OT WTE posts in the NHS departments covered by our enquiry, there were 77 WTE-established posts for unqualified staff, who were mainly called Helpers, Helper Technical Instructors or Technical Instructors. It was not possible to make a similar calculation for the local authorities, as there is no uniform grading structure; but what evidence there is suggests that well over half all those employed in work which would, broadly speaking, come under the rubric of occupational therapy were not qualified occupational therapists. There is no doubt, however, that without this cadre of unqualified staff the occupational therapy service in both the NHS and local government would be greatly impoverished, or indeed grind to a halt. Moreover it is clear that unqualified staff in occupational therapy departments are now, and in the future are more likely to be, a major source of recruitment of mature people to the profession. We decided, therefore, that it was vital to consider the relationships between the qualified and the unqualified in the provision of the service.

The work of the OT Helper and Technical Instructor

The College of Occupational Therapists defines the role of the Helper as 'to help to complement and provide continuity for the work of the qualified occupational therapist in aiding patients in their recovery', and it gives a broad job description in the following terms:

An Occupational Therapy Helper shall be a person appointed to work only under the guidance and supervision of a qualified occupational therapist to assist in carrying out duties, in the treatment of patients and in administrative functions.

Responsibilities

A. Personal duties

1. Is a member of a team and shares information with team members as directed.

2. Obtains information from patients/clients regarding their interests and skills.

3. Uses his/her acquired skills and techniques with groups and individual patients as directed.

4. Develops rapport with patients/clients to encourage their interest and participation in activity.

5. Observes general behaviour, ability and response of patients/clients and records the information as requested and reports to supervisor.

6. Assists with any community involvement under the guidance of professionally trained personnel.

B. Administrative

1. Must be aware of his/her responsibilities under HASWA in the local situation.

2. May be responsible for the maintenance of equipment and recommending the need for new items.

3. May be responsible for material stock and maintenance of stock levels.

4. May be responsible for maintenance of some Departmental records and rendering returns when requested.

5. May have other designated duties relating to particular needs of department or unit.

The College's definition of the role of Technical Instructor is similar, except that he/she is expected to hold a qualification in some trade or craft. There were some minor differences in the wording of the job description for the Technical Instructor, compared with that of the Helper, but virtually none in the list of their respective duties and administrative responsibilities.

The breadth of the job description is reflected in the wide range of activities in which, we learned, Helpers particularly, and Technical Instructors to a lesser extent, can be and are engaged. In some instances they appear to be, literally, maids of all work. Some Helpers work with patients under the supervision of the qualified occupational therapists, while others undertake typing, record-keeping, transport of people to day centres, routine delivery of apparatus to homes, servicing and repair of equipment, preparation of handicraft material – the list is endless. Local authorities, because they had for many years been obliged to provide aids and adaptations for those who needed them, had generally employed staff to make assessments of needs (some of whom also had the technical expertise to make and/or fit appliances) before they began to employ occupational therapists. Often such staff continue to be employed, and they are often paid on a salary scale which is higher than that of the Helper in NHS employment.

Some of the tasks undertaken by the unqualified, particularly work of the routine domestic kind, clearly require little in the way of training; many of the activities in which they engage, however, require either some degree of technical competence or 'morale maintenance' or 'man management' skills, which need both sensitive personal characteristics and the capacity to learn from experience on the job, as well as a good general level of educational attainment. Indeed there are undoubtedly some situations where Helpers and/or Technical Instructors are performing, at least for part of the time, the work expected of a qualified (and possibly experienced) occupational therapist. We do not doubt that many unqualified workers in such situations cope exceptionally well; however, many are aware that they lack the necessary basic training to work at the level which, unwittingly, may be demanded of them by managers, doctors or social workers.

In theory, as the definitions implied, Helpers and Technical Instructors are required to work *only* under the supervision of trained occupational therapists. In practice, however, as the evidence we received from many sources made clear, the failure to fill vacant posts for qualified OTs, or the filling of the only post in a small department by a young, inexperienced recent recruit, means that the work of the Helper or Technical Instructor is not merely essentially unsupervised; it is planned by such workers rather than by qualified occupational therapists. In the our view this happens frequently enough – especially in LASS departments, where the ratio of unqualified to qualified is much greater and where the former have had a longer history of employment than the latter – to make it understandable that service managers or members of other professions should often be unable to distinguish the qualified from the unqualified, or recognise the need for a proper complement of the former to lead and supervise the work.

Such situations would be less likely to arise had it been less difficult to fill vacancies for Basic grade qualified occupational therapists. In the NHS, for example, at 31 March 1988, 25.40% of established WTE posts for Basic grade occupational therapists were vacant, another 3.11% cut or frozen and only 71.49% filled. By contrast only 2.75% of Helpers WTE established posts were vacant, and 1.78% cut or frozen; 95.47% were filled. Moreover only 40.4% of the unqualified staff's vacant posts were known to have been vacant for more than three months, compared with 68.6% of the qualified staff's.

These situations reflect the problems associated with the growth of a profession which is at a comparatively early stage of its development, a topic which has been discussed at some length in Chapter 2. The problems are exacerbated, however, when the profession is charged with the responsibility of supervising those whose work had originally been identified and classified as technical, skilled manual or routine non-manual, but has since begun to acquire semi-professional status.

Resultant mismatches of experience and responsibility of this kind can lead to tensions in work relationships which are not easily resolved. It is to the credit of most occupational therapists – and their representative body – and also most of those working as Helpers and Technical Instructors and their Whitley Council spokesmen that the potential for tension and conflict has been so well contained and subordinated to the interests of patient welfare. Commonsense and a preparedness on all sides to compromise and adapt has nearly everywhere prevailed. This is particularly commendable at a time when lack of cooperativeness is increasingly and understandably advocated for professions – mostly those composed predominantly of women – which have fallen behind in salary and status, often because they have not been prepared to take what is now euphemistically known as 'industrial action'.

The Commission considered that the staffing situation in both NHS and LASS departments might be clearer to managers and other professional groups if the single designation 'Occupational Therapy Assistant' were to replace the present titles of Helper, Technical Instructor and others (especially in the local authority sector). These titles do not always represent accurately either the nature of the work or the degree of responsibility carried by any individual.

The ratio of qualified to unqualified work in occupational therapy

We are in no doubt that the future of occupational therapy depends upon a continuing supply of those who are called Technical Instructors or OT Helpers in the NHS, and a variety of names in LASS departments. It believes that occupational therapy, wherever it is practised, and in the fullest sense of the term, involves some work, of the kind already described in this chapter, which does not require a three-year course of diploma or degree standard to perform it adequately, as well as some work which does.

The ratio of qualified to unqualified *filled* WTE posts in the NHS, according to our own survey in 1988 was 1 to 0.9. For reasons already given, the Commission was not able to make a comparable calculation for the LASS sector. But the data it did obtain suggested that the ratio in that sector was likely to be more than reversed. That is, that there may have been less than 0.9 qualified to 1 unqualified.

In these circumstances we were not willing to make any definite statement about the desirable ratio in the future of qualified to unqualified staff across both employing sectors. Moreover we recognise that the ratio may need to vary *within* the NHS, depending upon the specialty. For example, we believe that the ratio of qualified to unqualified staff should be much higher in work with the mentally ill, where there is less scope for unqualified staff, than in work with the mentally handicapped. If, as is likely, the demand for occupational therapists in these two specialties increases disproportionately, the required ratios in each may bring about a balance, suggesting perhaps a long-term balanced ratio for occupational therapy in the NHS as a whole of 1 to 1. We were not able to explore this issue thoroughly, but believe that it should receive further serious attention from the College.

The College of Occupational Therapists itself has made its estimates of future staffing needs in the local authorities on the assumption that the correct ratio there would be of the order of 1 to 1.[1] We believe too that this ratio is

[1] 'Community occupational therapy. Future needs and numbers', COT 1984.

73

desirable. If it is to be achieved, however, it will be necessary to increase disproportionately the numbers of qualified occupational therapists in LASS departments, since at present there are more unqualified than qualified in work which is essentially occupational therapy.

In our view, an equalisation of the ratios of qualified to unqualified staff, as between the NHS and local authority employment sectors, would also be desirable on other grounds. They are that, in the light both of predictable demographic trends, including health and illness, and of the need for central government to implement the recommendations of the Griffiths Report,[2] or some such policy for community care, occupational therapy in the future should be building up its strength in the *community* services rather than in the hospitals. This is a theme to which the Commission adverts in the last chapter.

The education and training of Helpers and Technical Instructors

Systematic training for those recruited as Helpers or Technical Instructors to NHS occupational therapy departments or to the equivalent sections of LASS departments has evolved only recently in piecemeal fashion. As occupational therapists themselves began to recognise the need for some systematic instruction of their unqualified Helpers, the College's Education Board took upon itself the task of devising an in-service course of 216 hours for Helpers. It is run by District or Head Occupational Therapists. It is not everywhere available, and some occupational therapists have not put such

[2] R. Griffiths, *Community Care: Agenda for Action*, HMSO London, 1988.

courses high on the list of their priorities. Participation is voluntary, and not a condition of employment, although those who take the courses do so in their employers' time. Completion of the course carries a certificate of attendance, but attracts no pay differential or other official recognition. Hence it carries little status. There are relatively few opportunities to take this in-service course or a comparable one for the non-qualified equivalents in LASS departments of NHS Helpers and Technical Instructors.

We were told that many of those recruited to the post of Helper or Technical Instructor, often after family-building, or on a mid-life change of career decision, are not particularly ambitious or career-minded. They regard their work as a nine-to-five job, pleasurable in itself, but not one in which they want to advance, especially if it involves further study. Nevertheless we believe that every individual who joins an OT department in either the NHS or LASS should have the opportunity to acquire a qualification at an appropriate level of NCVQ I-IV, with a salary reflecting her or his level of qualification and experience.

By no means all those who have joined occupational therapy departments, however, have been content to coast along, without seeking to further their career prospects. Whatever their motives and ambitions on initial recruitment, a significant minority has become intrigued with the job, anxious to learn more, and to accept more responsibility. In short these OT auxiliaries have sought the opportunity to progress to full professional status, and in some, but by no means all, areas some enthusiastic OT educationalists and practitioners have designed courses to enable Helpers to do just this. There are courses in Essex, Crawley, Bristol and Brent, and perhaps elsewhere too. They are organised on the basis of a day-and-a-half study release per week, over a four year period. There are academic and other tests of attainment, and those who pass are awarded a qualification recognised by the occupational therapists' professional body and then placed on the profession's register.

We understand that if such courses were available throughout the country, so that many more Helpers could take them, it would meet a demand and help to recruit a stable labour force of more mature individuals likely to give, on average, as long professional service, as does the intake into the present training colleges of students of school-leaving age. We thought that more encouragement should be given by the College of Occupational Therapists to such courses, which, at present, rely entirely for their establishment and running on local initiative.

Finally we did consider, if only to dismiss it fairly quickly, the desirability of including OT Helpers in a common core basic training for 'generic care assistants' who would do everything for a handicapped person that a caring relative would do. There may well be a case for such an occupational group, but this is not the place to discuss such a development. However, if such a course were to be instituted, we felt that instruction in some of the skills and understanding which the OT Helper needs should be included in it. However, OT Helpers, in our view, will need a higher level of qualification than that of the projected generic care assistant.

6

Industrial Relations and Professional Status

The existing representation, recognition and negotiating arrangements for the profession are complex. They are partly explained by the fact that since 1978 the British Association of Occupational Therapists has had to conform to the new industrial relations legislation, and to set itself up as a certificated trade union. That left a requirement for a separate body to function as an educational charity. The College of Occupational Therapists was formed as a wholly-owned subsidiary of BAOT and carries out all the functions typically seen in a body responsible for validating training or educational courses, controlling qualification and promoting knowledge and standards.

We asked ourselves three main questions. How does BAOT represent its members? How well does it perform as a trade union? Are there any alternative arrangements which would clearly improve its role and functions? Occupational therapy is a profession whose members have shown little interest in, or enthusiasm for, industrial relations, let alone engagement in industrial action. It has even considered that industrial action would be professionally inappropriate. We record that much, neither in the spirit of compliment nor of criticism.

77

Members have probably, on the whole, arrived at a sensible evaluation of their own industrial power among the various groups of employees in local authority employment, the National Health Service and elsewhere. However great their dissatisfactions at their terms and conditions of public employment, they have preferred to rely on remedies of persuasion and argument. This, to date, has not perceptibly accentuated recruitment difficulties, resignations and a seeming reluctance to return to the profession. This is in any event a profession which, in numerical terms, forms a very small proportion of the total staffing complement of the NHS and the local authorities; as such its negotiating impact is correspondingly minimal.

Most occupational therapists work in the NHS: just over 5,000. Nearly 1,000 work for local authorities, and just over 500 work in the private sector. Between 80% and 85% of all registered occupational therapists are members of BAOT. However, BAOT has attracted less than a fifth of Helpers and Technical Instructors to associate membership. In the list of Professions Allied to Medicine it ranks in numbers qualified and registered as follows:

MLSO	20,134
Physiotherapists	19,780
Radiographers	15,160
OCCUPATIONAL THERAPISTS	9,306
Chiropodists	6,142
Dietitians	2,584
Orthoptists	966

BAOT has developed its own structure of committees to ventilate and formulate industrial relations policies. In the NHS occupational therapists' interests in pay are pursued by BAOT's own representations to the Review Body. It participates in preliminary meetings with the Federation of Professional Organisations so that a coherent stance can be offered to the Staff Side. Conditions of service in the NHS, e.g. holidays and hours of work, are determined through the Whitley Council machinery, in which BAOT also plays a full part. In the NHS, BAOT is encouraging the development of a steward network, one for each district and one for each region to represent more senior staff.

In the local authority field, there has been no prospect that BAOT would be recognised. By contrast with the NHS (Review Body) each local authority thus can decide for itself the pay and conditions of occupational therapists. In England and Wales it is not surprising to find considerable differences in pay, grading and career structure. There are differences between local authorities, and between local authorities and the NHS. The local authority recognition issue presented BAOT with a severe problem. The only course seemed to be some sort of association with one of the five unions recognised in local government. NALGO did not present an attractive trade union to occupational therapists. Moreover double membership would not have been possible. Only recently (in 1985) an agreement was concluded with MATSA (Managerial, Administrative, Technical and Supervisory Association), which is a section of the General Municipal Boilermakers and Allied Trades Union. This enables occupational therapists to apply for joint membership. MATSA negotiates on their behalf and BAOT can put to MATSA arguments on pay and conditions.

The working of the BAOT/MATSA relationship is naturally a frequent item on the agenda of BAOT's Salaries and Industrial Relations Committee. A trade union needs to keep abreast of the general aspirations of its members. Suggestions that a new union should be formed, comprising all or some of the professions listed above, would run ahead of the wishes of most occupational therapists. Even if this could be achieved, there is no guarantee that the result would be greater bargaining leverage with the employers. If the professions of physiotherapy and occupational therapy were to combine, a new combined union might then make sense. But mergers and formal institutional changes, which engender their own misgivings among members, capture support only if they follow in the wake of other major changes made for widely-accepted professional reasons. There is also the obvious point that the present political climate hardly favours the creation of new unions.

BAOT and the College have made considerable efforts to respond appropriately to the wishes of members, and the Commission, in the circumstances, has no suggestions for internal structural change. Occupational therapists will wish that the recent BAOT/MATSA agreement and its workings be kept under the closest possible scrutiny. We urge that this surveillance should continue. Unions are only as effective as their members. Much depends on the willingness of individual occupational therapists to contribute more of their own time and energy. In their dealings with the Federation of Professional Organisations and the Pay Review Body we have concluded that the contribution of OT members has been impressive and astute.

Two minor matters deserve mention. First, the profession, as this Report constantly observes, is predominantly female. BAOT should, therefore, be peculiarly responsive to problems on the Equal Opportunities front, and be prepared to pursue vigorously any matter affecting members or putative members, which relates to this cultural issue. Second, the *British Journal of Occupational Therapy*, published monthly, does not carry any items on salaries or conditions of service for fear that the registered charitable status of the College might be endangered, but it could usefully carry loose inserts from time to time, drawing attention to issues of employment conditions.

The future role of BAOT

As for securing greater recognition or bargaining power for the profession through some different form of trade union machinery, we do not contemplate any realistic alternative to that already in place. We do suggest, however, that, within the present structure of BAOT and COT, it is possible for both bodies to be more vigorous in formulating and pursuing the aims and objectives of the profession. It is possible to separate out two main approaches to the aims toward objectives:

1. The trade union approach aims to raise the standing of the profession, by forcing it up the ladder of salary rewards through collective bargaining or other industrial pressures.
2. The learned society approach aims to raise the standing of the profession, by increasing its esteem in the eyes of the general public and other competing professions.

In practice the actions which the two discrete approaches require overlap and, therefore, also overlap the notional spheres of influence of BAOT and COT. But, as long as this is recognised, it will be no obstacle. A brief description, outlining some of the actions which could be taken in pursuit of the approaches might be as follows:

The first could be done by increasing the effectiveness and efficiency of the operations of the professions and by demonstrating that increase by means of evaluation and monitoring studies of performance, particularly that of added value. For example, it is possible that if there were more occupational therapists there would be fewer demands on the Health Service, because more people would become or remain independent of it. This proposition is susceptible to objective verification. The results can also be expressed in terms of added value. Systematic attitudinal studies should also be regularly carried out as a means of 'marketing' the profession to neighbouring professions, to the NHS apparatus and to the public in general.

The second approach is best achieved by raising the intellectual horizons of the profession and its members. This is done successfully by other professions in a variety of ways – from highly visible promotional activities, such as national and international conferences, symposia and meetings, to strictly educational activities such as research, study leave and post-experience qualifying courses.

In both instances there should be annually agreed targets and appraisals of the results of these kind of exercises. It would also be wise to encourage personal appraisal procedures to reach every OT, Helper and Instructor, so that the profession is seen to be vitally interested in professional standards, and in control of them.

Accompanying these overall activities there needs to be a constant exhortation to individual occupational therapists to seek every way to develop self-esteem and display it extensively. It needs to be based on vigorous performance, fearlessly and rigorously evaluated and effectively made known. To parody the still valid words from the past, the best public relations advice in these circumstances follows the storyboard – 'By their actions ye shall know them'.

7

Conclusions and Recommendations

While we were still deliberating, the Government produced its policies for the future of the acute sector of the National Health Service in the form of a White Paper (*Working for Patients: Caring for the 1990s*), which contains radical proposals for both hospital management and the general practice sector.

As we come to the end of our investigation and prepare our report it is still not clear how far the Government may modify its proposals in the light of reactions to the White Paper. Moreover, although there have been well-informed rumours, the Government has not yet indicated, officially, how far it proposes to implement the recommendations of the Griffiths Report (*Care in the Community: Agenda for Action, 1988*) or make other proposals affecting the long-term care of elderly and disabled people, which will have even greater significance for the future of occupational therapy than the proposals for the acute sector.

In these uncertain circumstances we feel that we are not in a position to make any precise proposals as to how the profession can best implement all our recommendations, let alone respond to the challenges implied in the Government's own proposals. The status of occupational therapists in their assessment and treatment of patients must be fully recognised; and their skills fully employed both in the acute sector of the National Health Service and in helping the chronically sick and disabled in the community.

This concluding chapter thus consists mainly of a reiteration of recommendations made in earlier chapters. Here, those recommendations are summarised under seven, albeit overlapping, headings. We urge all members of the profession and those concerned with the planning and management of health and social services to read the socio-economic analysis contained in the first two chapters, since it provides the overall justification for the recommendations, as well as the subsequent chapters which provide detailed reasons for them.

Recommendations

Numbers and norms

The College of Occupational Therapists should:

1.1 aim for an 80% expansion in the number of qualified OTs by the end of the century (Chapter 2, page 39);

1.2 put pressure upon Government to establish nation-ally applicable norms for posts for qualified OTs and their assistants (Chapter 2, page 25);

1.3 revise and update its own norms which should be for combined NHS and LASS authorities (Chapter 2, page 38);

1.4 consider afresh the ratio of qualified to unqualified staff in both NHS and LASS employment (Chapter 5, page 73);

1.5 reduce the numbers of trained occupational therapists leaving the profession altogether, by providing greater help to young Basic Grade OTs, and by instituting or improving re-induction courses for re-entrants (Chapter 2, page 37);

1.6 investigate the discrepancy between the numbers qualifying annually and the number of Basic grade recruits in post (Chapter 2, page 40).

Deployment

The College of Occupational Therapists should:

2.1 accelerate the pace of change, already taking place, towards a re-deployment of occupational therapists to work in the community, rather than in hospitals (Chapter 2, page 39)

2.2 examine rigorously procedures and practices to ensure that qualified occupational therapists do not undertake work which could be undertaken by other less highly trained staff, and ensure that untrained staff are not left to undertake work for which they are not properly prepared (Chapter 3, page 48).

Recruitment

The College of Occupational Therapists should:

3.1 continue and intensify present methods of acquainting school career officers and others with the attractions of occupational therapy as a caring profession (Chapter 4, page 58);

3.2 sustain present entry requirements for school leaver recruits (Chapter 4, page 59);

3.3 continue to suspend minimum entry requirements for mature applicants and to take into account their experience and motivation (Chapter 4, page 59);

3.4 redouble efforts to attract graduates from a variety of disciplines and continue to offer them accelerated qualifying courses (Chapter 4, page 60).

Preparation

The College of Occupational Therapists should:

4.1 give serious consideration to a degree of specialisation in either the physical or the psychiatric field in the second half or third year of the basic course, after a common core which should be both theoretical and practical (Chapter 4, page 61);

4.2 establish closer relations with universities and/or polytechnics to enable fuller use to be made of a wider range of expertise in basic courses (Chapter 4, page 64);

4.3 encourage full-time teachers to return to practice posts periodically to maintain their touch, and consider ways of keeping closer contact with field supervisors (Chapter 4, page 62);

4.4 give greater priority in some districts to the provision of in-service courses to enable suitable helpers to qualify (Chapter 5, page 75).

7. Conclusions and Recommendations

Qualifying standards

The College of Occupational Therapists should:

5.1 enter into negotiations promptly with the Council for National Academic Awards (CNAA) and selected universities with a view to validating the profession's present qualifying credential (the Diploma) as a degree of equivalent status to those at present awarded in Scottish and English universities (Chapter 4, page 62);

5.2 institute a further year of supervised work following qualification, which must be completed satisfactorily, before full registration as an occupational therapist (Chapter 4, page 61).

Negotiating machinery

The College of Occupational Therapists should:

6.1 with BAOT formulate more positively their aims and objectives and pursue them rigorously in the negotiating bodies of both the NHS and Local Government (Chapter 6, page 81);

6.2 seek to obtain more opportunities for senior occupational therapists in LASS to be considered for management posts at all levels (Chapter 3, page 55).

Professional enhancement

The College of Occupational Therapists should:

7.1 review once gain the advantages and disadvantages

of joining forces with physiotherapists to form a single therapy profession, with post-qualification specialisation (Chapter 3, page 50);

7.2 keep under regular consideration the desirability of finding a new name for the profession which would more accurately reflect its present knowledge, skills and accomplishments, and cast off lingering, derogatory stereotypes derived from its amateur origins (Chapter 1, page 17);

7.3 seek to validate the profession's claims to professional status by devising ways of measuring and monitoring the effectiveness and efficiency of practices, procedures and organisational arrangements (Chapter 3, page 46, and Chapter 6, page 81);

7.4 encourage OT units to set agreed targets for themselves and for every member annually and to appraise performance in their light (Chapter 6, page 82);

7.5 authorise attitudinal studies among fellow professionals and client groups, as a means of 'marketing', creating and maintaining a buoyant demand for the profession's services (Chapter 6, page 82);

7.6 raise the profession's public profile by initiating and holding multi-disciplinary conferences, seminars and workshops to consider common health and welfare objectives and the means of achieving them (Chapter 6, page 82).

By and large, we are not recommending any drastic change of course for occupational therapists. Indeed many of our recommendations to the profession are to reinforce decisions already taken by it or under its active consideration. Needless to say, we believe that, whatever changes take place in the context in which occupational therapists will have to function in the future, the profession and its patients and clients will undoubtedly benefit if the recommendations are implemented.

Whatever the outcome of the Government's discussion on the future of the National Health Service and on the Griffiths Report, an early opportunity to be in the forefront of community care presents itself to occupational therapists, who should prepare themselves for the developing opportunities in the field of community care. It might be possible, for example, for a National Occupational Therapy Service to be organised which could provide appropriate services on contract to Health Service and Social Services Authorities, to independent providers of services and to individuals.

The Commission's overriding recommendation to the College of Occupational Therapy is to prepare its members for an exciting future in the practice of occupational therapy. In the process of achieving that object occupational therapy will cease to be the submerged profession of today. Tomorrow occupational therapists should emerge as major practitioners in community care.

Appendix A: The Commission

Members

Professor Eva Alberman, Professor of Clinical Epidemiology, The London Hospital Medical College

Mr Louis Blom-Cooper QC, Chairman, Press Council; Chairman, Mental Health Act Commission

Professor Roger Dyson, Professor of Adult and Continuing Education, University of Keele. (Professor Dyson was unable to act as a Commissioner after July 1988 due to administrative commitments at the University of Keele.)

Sir Graham Hills, Vice-Chancellor and Principal, Strathclyde University

Professor Margot Jefferys, Professor Emeritus of the Sociology of Medicine, University of London

Mrs Patricia Marshall, Chief Nursing Officer, City and Hackney Health Authority

Miss Mary Mason, Former Director of Social Services, Bolton Metropolitan Borough Council

Mr Hugh Pierce, Former Assistant Controller, Staff Administration, BBC

Dr Douglas Price, General Practitioner

Mr Brian Roycroft, Director of Social Services, Newcastle-upon-Tyne; President, Association of Directors of Social Services 1988-1989

Professor Philip Seager, Director, Health Advisory Service; Professor of Psychiatry, University of Sheffield

Appendix A

Mr Peter Wood, Chairman, Huddersfield Health Authority
Andrew Young, Professor Emeritus of Mathematics, University of Ulster

Written submissions and oral evidence

Argyll & Clyde Health Board. Merchiston Hospital
Armistead Child Development Centre. Elizabeth N. Fairgrieve
Ashby (Ann), Chairman Trent Regional Group & Rotherham District OT
Ass. Professions for Mentally Handicapped People

BAOT. Stephanie Correia – Chairman, Salaries & Industrial Relations
Bangour Village Hospital. Lily Jeffrey
BASW
Belfast: Visit by P.E. Wood
Bloomsbury Rheumatology Unit. Michael Shipley
Bristol & Weston H.A. Farleigh Hospital
British Dietetic Ass. John Grigg
British Medical Association
British Orthopaedic Ass. B. McKibbin
British Paediatric Association. Dr T.L. Chambers
British Psychological Society. Colin Newman
British Red Cross. Medical Aid Dept. Leicestershire
British Soc. for Rheumatology
Buckinghamshire Health Authorities

Cambridgeshire Social Services Dept.
Cardiological Rehabilitation. Charing Cross Experience
Centre for Policy on Ageing
Chartered Society of Physiotherapy. Penelope Robinson
Chest, Heart & Stroke Ass. Sir David Atkinson
Christ Church College Dept of OT
Claybury Hospital, Essex
Clwyd Co. Council. Mrs W.P. Edwards
College of Ripon & York St. John. P.H. Juffs
College of Speech Therapists: Margaret Edwards and Dominic Wyseman
COT. Statement on OT Referral
Council for Professions Supplementary to Medicine. Miss B.U. Folkard
Council of Heads of OT Training Schools
Currie (Mrs Edwina) MP

The Commission

Department of Health & Social Security. John M. Rodgers
Disabled Living Foundation. Aids & Equipment Centre, Peggy Jay
 and Elizabeth Fanshaw
Disablement Services Authority. W.V. James
Doncaster Health Authority. Mrs Rachel Lund
Dorset House School of OT, Oxford
Dudley Metropolitan Borough. Social Services Dept. E.A. Askew
Dundee Royal Infirmary. Malcolm McInnes

East Cumbria H.A. Garlands Hospital
Edwards (Mrs), Clwyd.
Edwards (Margaret). Speech Therapist

Fielding (Miss K.M.) Dip COT SROT
Fife Regional Council
Friern Hospital, London

Gardner (Dr P.)
Garlands Hospital. R.A. Lambert
Gartnavel Royal Hospital. Mrs Fiona Gordon
Glasgow School of OT. Mrs B.R. Hudson
Greater Glasgow Health Board
Guy's Hospital. Newcomen Centre. Christina Gericke

Hall (Jean) DipCOT, SR, MBAOT
Health Visitors Association. Shirley Goodwin
Hertfordshire Social Services. North Area
Highland Health Board
Holderness Community. Mental Health Team. S. Phipps

Islington Council Social Services Dept. A.M. Gibbs

John Radcliffe Hospital. Mrs Rosemary Bowden

Leicester Frith Hospital
Leicester Social Services Dept.
Leicestershire County Council Referrals' Report
Leicestershire County Council Service Profile
Liverpool Institute of Higher Education (OT Dept.) Rosemary Barnit
Liverpool Social Services
London Boroughs OT Managers Group. Gillian Stoddart
London School of OT. West London Inst. Higher Education

Mackenzie (Alice).
Maidstone Heath Authority. Mrs U. Lakhera

Appendix A

Mersey Regional Group of OTs
Mertens (H.A.), Senior OT, Buckinghamshire
Mid-Essex District OT
Mid-Glamorgan Health Authority
Middlesborough Gen. Hospital. Dept. of Rehabilitation. Susan Al-
    Bassam
Milton Keynes Health Authority
Moorhaven Hospital. OT Dept. Christine Taylor and others
Mortimer (Jess)
MPAG. OT Staffing Structures & Skill Mix Study

National Mobility Centre
Noble (Mrs Jean)
North East Essex H.A. St Mary's Hospital. Mrs. J. Castle
Northern Health & Social Services Board, Antrim
Northern Ireland Committee COT
Northern Ireland/Scotland. Report by A. Young
Norwich H.A. Hales Hospital
Norwich H.A. Whitlingham Hospital
Nottinghamshire Co. Council Social Services. Peter Finch

Oxfordshire Health Authority. John Radcliffe Hospital
Oxfordshire Regional Health Authority. Tom Plant

PAM. Second Report 1985
Parkinson's Disease Society
Pitts (Joanna). OT Officer

Queen Margaret College, Edinburgh. Morag Stott

RADAR. Leslie Browne
Redbridge Ass. for Handicapped People
Redbridge Health Authority. Nicholas Darling
Ridout (Mrs), Basingstoke
Rochdale Metropolitan Borough Council
Royal College of General Practitioners
Royal College of Physicians. Faculty of Community Medicine. J.A.
    Anderson
Royal College of Surgeons
Royal Edinburgh Hospital
Royal National Institute for the Blind
Royal National Institute for the Deaf
Royal Society of Medicine. R.N. Thomson
Royal Victoria Hospital, Edinburgh – Virginia Hanrahan

Scottish Central Regional Group of OTs. Christine Duncan

The Commission

Sheffield Health Authority
Slade Hospital, Oxford
Society of Community Medicine
South Glamorgan H.A. University Hosp. of Wales
South Glamorgan H.A. Training brochure
South Tees H.A. Dept of Rehabilitation
Southampton & South West Hants Regional Authority
Special Children Therapy Campaign
Spoors (Brenda)
Squire (C.), London
St Andrew's Hospital, Norwich
St Andrew's Hospital. Elizabeth Cracknell. Head of OT Dept.
St George's Hospital. (Paediatric. Interest. People). Ms Beryl Steeden
St Loye's School of OT
St Martin's Hospital
Strathclyde Regional Council. Dorothy Gormlie
Swann (Sylvia) Dip.COT SROT

Tameside Health Authority. Jennifer Creek
Tayside Health Board. Armistead Centre, Dundee
Tone Vale Hospital, Somerset
Trent Regional Authority. Betty Zuger

Walsall Health Authority
Wandsworth Council Social Services Dept.
Wanstead Hospital
Welsh School of OT
Wessex Regional Health Authority
West London Institute of Higher Education
White (Susan Mary) Dip.COT SROT.
Whitlingham Hospital. Mrs E. Bumthrey
Woodlanders PSA and LINK Hands

Visits made by Members of the Commission

12 February 1988	COT Council Meeting, London	Mary Mason
February 1988	Univ. of Ulster Dept. of OT	Andrew Young
10 March 1988	Dept of Cardiology, Charing Cross Hospital	Douglas Price
7 April 1988	St John's Hospital, Chelmsford	Douglas Price
13-15 April 1988	COT Seminar, Warwick	Mary Mason
		Andrew Young
		Margot Jefferys
		Philip Seager
		Douglas Price

95

Appendix A

19 April 1988	Northern Ireland Committee of COT	Andrew Young Philip Seager Peter Wood
2 May 1988	Queen Margaret's College, Edinburgh	Mary Mason Graham Hills Andrew Young
23 June 1988	St Loyes College, Exeter	Philip Seager
29 June 1988	St Peter's Hospital, Chertsey	Douglas Price
30 June 1988	Mrs Mitchell Heal, Staff & Students of Dorset House	Margot Jefferys Douglas Price
1 July 1988	Ottershaw Geriatric Day Hospital, Surrey	Douglas Price

National vocational qualifications

Level I

Occupational competence in performing a range of tasks under supervision.

Level II

Occupational competence in performing a wider, more demanding range of tasks with limited supervision.

Level III

Occupational competence required for satisfactory responsible performance in a defined occupation or range of jobs.

Level IV

Competence to design and specify defined tasks, products and processes and to accept responsibility for the work of others.

Appendix B

Survey of 1987-1988 Staffing Levels
for Occupational Therapy Departments
in the United Kingdom

Paper prepared by Professor E. Alberman
with the help of Ms Anita Horwich
and Ms Sheila Williams

Contents

Appendix B

Annexes:

1. This survey was specifically undertaken within the context of the inquiries being conducted by the Independent Commission on Occupational Therapy that was established in November 1987 under the chairmanship of Mr Louis Blom Cooper QC, with the mandate 'To review the existing and future demands upon, and the available manpower resources of, the profession of Occupational Therapy, having regard to the social, demographic and epidemiological trends into the twenty-first century, and to report with recommendations'. The Commission recognised that it would not be able to carry out this mandate effectively unless it had at its disposal statistics on current occupational therapy (OT) staffing levels throughout the country that were both accurate and comprehensive. It also felt that it would be desirable for the necessary analysis to be prepared by a qualified person who is not directly associated either with the OT profession or with any of the government bodies responsible for health care

* The tables in Annexes 2 and 3 are taken from *Key population and vital statistics 1987* (HMSO 1989).

100

management, and who would preferably be a member of the Commission.

Organisation and scope of the survey

2. The collection of the required data was placed in the hands of the College of Occupational Therapists (COT). The College sent out questionnaires to the heads of the individual OT Departments in both the NHS and the Local Authority Social Services (LASSs) but it was decided that the survey should not try to cover the available OT manpower resources that exist outside the health and social services, and personnel in private practice[1] or working as teachers in the various training establishments are therefore omitted.

3. During discussions with COT it was agreed that the questionnaire circulated to the NHS Departments would be simultaneously used by the College as a basis for preparing material for the annual submission made by the British Association of Occupational Therapists (BAOT) to the Government Pay Review Body for Professions Allied to Medicine. It is important to note that as a consequence the types of questions inserted in the form were required to be compatible with the equivalent questionnaires being sent out by the representative bodies of the other PAMs in connection with the 1989 Pay Review. For this reason no changes could be made to any of the wordings used for determining the categories of data requested, although substantial adjustments to the format of the questionnaire originally presented by the College did have to

[1] BAOT statistics indicate that at end October 1987 524 of its members were in the private sector; membership of BAOT is estimated to be between 80-85% of all registered OTs.

be introduced in order to facilitate the subsequent computer processing.

Coverage of the questionnaire

4. The information sought was to apply to all staff posts within each OT Department for the year period 1.4.87 – 31.3.88.

5. As shown in the two sample pages – one taken from the NHS questionnaire and the other from the LASS questionnaire – attached at Annex 1, the OT in charge of the Department was asked to enter on a single line the following information per post: title and grade, the date the post was created, the number of hours per week assigned to the post, the number of weeks the post may have remained vacant or otherwise unfilled, whether an unfilled post had been permanently cut or temporarily frozen, the functional allocation of hours of work, reasons for a staff member leaving a post, and the intake and source of any new recruit to a post.

6. It can be seen that the two questionnaires were virtually identical except in respect to the eight specified functional areas of work. In the NHS form these were designated as: Acute Medicine, Acute Surgery, Geriatrics, Paediatrics, the Mentally Ill, the Mentally Handicapped, Community Work, and Administration. In the LASS form the specified areas were: the Adult Physically Handicapped, Mental Health, the Mentally Handicapped, Children, Day Care, Residential Care, Housing, and Management. Allowance was also made in both forms for indicating unspecified 'Other' areas of work.

Response rates

(a) from NHS Departments

7. Of the 212 OT Departments established in UK hospitals only 14 failed to reply, which is equivalent to a response rate of 93.4%. However, six of the completed questionnaires were not returned in time for inclusion, so that the actual survey is based on a response rate of 91.0%.

8. The regional distribution of the 20 Departments thus omitted from the survey is as follows: 1 from Trent, 1 from East Anglia, 3 from NW Thames, 1 from NE Thames, 1 from SE Thames, 1 from SW Thames, 1 from S. Western, 1 from W. Midlands, 3 from N. Western, 2 from Wales, 5 from Scotland. Annex 2 giving 1987 population estimates for each of the UK's Districts/Areas shows that the proportion of total UK population represented in the 192 Districts/Areas covered by the survey was the same as the overall response rate from the OT Departments, 91%.

(b) from LASS Departments

9. The response rate on the LASS side was not quite so rewarding. Of the 128 Authorities contacted, 95 sent in replies. But since nine of these Authorities stated that they do not employ OTs, this meant that only 86 actually completed the questionnaire, equivalent to a response of 74%. All the LASS contacted are listed in Annex 3.

Appendix B

Regional framework for the survey

(a) for the NHS data

10. NHS OT Departments are computed as being distributed among the following Health Regions: the 14 Regions within England, plus Wales, N. Ireland, and Scotland. In other words, although Scotland has its own separate Health Regions – Scotland Northern, Central, Eastern and Western, each administered by a Board equivalent to England's Regional Health Authorities (RHAs) – it is treated here as a single unit.

11. In addition to the 17 Health Regions indicated, the survey also covered the OT Departments maintained in specialist graduate hospitals that are located in London but take patients from all over the United Kingdom, and which are collectively managed by the Special Health Authority (Special HA). Special HA is regarded as having equivalent status to the RHAs, even though it does not serve a local population and is therefore outside the regional organisation of the health service.

(b) for the LASS data

12. The 128 Local Authorities contacted included the various Metropolitan Boroughs and County Councils in England and Wales as well as the Scottish Regional Councils' Social Work Departments. In the case of N. Ireland, though, where the health and social services are fully integrated under the management of four subregional Boards, no administrative distinction is drawn between OTs working in NHS hospitals and at the community level and all these staff were therefore

already covered by the replies received in response to the
NHS questionnaire.

13. It will be appreciated that there could be no question
of extracting statistics on the basis of the regional
breakdown which was used for the NHS material. Not
only would N. Ireland have had to be omitted, but in most
cases the geographic area covered by specific LASSs is
not coterminous with that placed under the management
of a given RHA. Nor, of course, is there any direct
administrative link between the LASSs and RHAs.

Differentiation of staff posts

(a) in the NHS

14. Depending on the size of a given OT Department,
there may be up to a total of nine categories of
established Posts: the four categories for professionally
qualified OTs recognised by the Whitley Council – titled
District, Head, Senior and Basic; and five categories for
unqualified staff – designated in the questionnaire as
Helper TI,[2] Helper, TI, Therapist, and Other (i.e.
secretaries, clerks etc). Allowance was made in the form
for distinguishing the 13 recognised seniority grades
within the Whitley Council grading structure (e.g. Heads
I-IV, Senior I & II). However, in order to avoid excessive
complexity in the presentation of the statistical analysis,
it was decided to confine the differentiation of staff posts
simply to the nine categories indicated. This explains
why the term 'category' has been used throughout the
following text instead of the more usual term 'grade',

2 TI stands for Technical Instructor.

since the latter implies a level of differentiation that has in fact been excluded from the survey.

(b) in the LASS

15. The LASSs do not apply a uniform grading structure for the OTs in their employment; while some Authorities may have introduced the Whitley Council categories and grades, the majority have adopted their own independent systems which, moreover, may not even always draw a clear distinction between qualified and unqualified staff. In consequence, although most of the replies to the questionnaire duly inserted the title and grade of posts as requested, it was impossible to establish categories for the statistical analysis which would be applicable to all the different LASS structures. Hence the OTs employed in each Authority surveyed have had to be treated as an undifferentiated staff group.

Usage of terms

(i) 'vacant' post

16. An unfilled established post is one which may have been cut or frozen or have become vacant because no one has replaced a departing member of staff. For the purposes of the present survey a post is defined as 'vacant' if it was not cut or frozen but had no incumbent at 31.3.88. This definition is not the same as that used by the DHSS which specifically does not count a post as being officially 'vacant' until after 12 weeks. The organising bodies representing the various PAMs take the view that the DHSS's interpretation is both unrealistic and misleading. At the same time they have

recognised that merely to indicate that a post happens to be vacant at a given date is equally unsatisfactory. They therefore agreed that they should all include a 'number of weeks vacant' column in their respective questionnaire relating to the 1989 Pay Review.[3] The survey is thus able to show data on posts that had been vacant for more than 12 weeks at 31.3.88, compatible with the DHSS definition, as well as on vacancies specifically on this date.

(ii) 'established' post

17. Again for the purpose of this survey every post listed was regarded as 'established', including those originally established but subsequently cut or temporarily frozen because of lack of resources or because no applicant found as well as vacant posts. It appears that RHAs count as established only the posts which are filled together with those labelled vacant, but this has the effect of hiding resource cuts which may have been introduced during the year period.

Preparation of statistical material

18. Although in most surveys applying to the health field statistical data is usually expressed solely in terms of whole time equivalents (WTEs) – which are the number of hours assigned to a particular staff member or functional area divided by 36 – rather than in terms of full-time (36 hours per week) 'Posts', it was felt that it might be useful to prepare parallel tables using the two sets of terms. This will permit detailed study at a later stage, to be undertaken perhaps by COT or relevant NHS

---

[3] For previous Pay Reviews, only some of the PAMs had in fact submitted data on the number of weeks a posts remained vacant.

management bodies, of the numbers of part-time staff employed in the different OT Departments (the closer the two sets of figures are in any given pair of parallel tables, the fewer the numbers of part-time staff employed). In the present paper, however, with only a few exceptions all the various findings described have been related to WTEs, in conformity with customary practice.

Validity check

19. For one Health Region for which there was a full return, NE Thames, it proved possible to compare the survey returns with those collected for the same date by the RHA manpower team. After adjustment to ensure that the same definitions were used, the numbers of filled posts for both qualified and unqualified staff from the two sources were within 5% of each other, and the numbers of filled qualified posts were almost identical. There was a slightly greater difference between the survey and the regional data on established posts but even this was within 10%. The RHA manpower manager considered the comparison to be satisfactorily close, well within the margins of expected differences. It is hoped to carry out similar comparisons for other Regions.

Analysis of principal findings

20. All the tables prepared for the purposes of the survey can be made available on request but, as will be appreciated, it would be too cumbersome to attach the complete set to this paper. The most detailed findings are those that relate to the NHS material, but comparisons from the LASS data are given wherever possible.

21. Since so many numbers have perforce had to be

incorporated into this section of the paper, for easier
reading the WTE totals as presented in the written text
are frequently given in rounded figures rather than in the
decimal numbers shown on the actual tables. It must also
be pointed out that whenever the word 'post/s' appears
without an initial capital it is being used only in the sense
of a general job position and not in the strict meaning of
the term 'Post/s' signifying the full-time establishments
which formed one of the basic determinants in computing
the tables.

Numbers of established posts/WTEs included in the survey

22. The information contained in the responses to the
NHS questionnaire received by the due date covered
13,877 established Posts. However, statistics for 262 of
these had to be excluded from the analysis either because
of incomplete data given or because they were
established after 1.4.88. Thus the number of established
Posts analysed in the present survey is 13,615,
corresponding to 11,426 WTEs.

23. For the LASS material, the replies received covered a
total establishment of 1,922 Posts, corresponding to
1,669 WTEs. The LASS WTEs can be estimated to
increase the overall total of OT hours available
throughout the United Kingdom by approximately 15%,
after correction for non-responding districts.

Distribution of established posts/WTEs

24. As at 31.3.88 the 13,615 Posts/11,426 WTEs established in the 192 NHS OT Departments surveyed were
distributed between the 9 staff categories as follows:

Appendix B

Qualified NHS Staff	Posts	WTEs
District OTs	173	169.1
Heads	1,213	1,167.3
Seniors	4,149	3,479.2
Basic	1,752	1,623.4
Sub Total	7,287	6,439.0
Unqualified NHS Staff		
Helper TIs	1,689	1,406.7
Helpers	3,225	2,437.8
TIs	799	724.8
Therapists	217	162.9
Others	398	254.9
Sub Total	6,328	4,987.2
Total All NHS Staff	13,615	11,426.1

25. The regional distribution of established WTEs for all staff categories is shown in Table 1 where it can be seen that totals range from over 900 WTEs in Trent and W. Midlands to middle levels of between 633-864 for 8 Regions and between 483-514 for 6 Regions, with N. Ireland at the bottom of the scale with 317. Special HA with only 58 WTEs is obviously of an entirely different order.

26. It is clear, though, that these figures cannot form an adequate basis for drawing meaningful comparisons until the Regions are related to their respective population figures. Table 2 shows, in the third column, a national distribution of 0.22 WTEs per 1,000 UK population. The regional distribution of WTEs per 1,000 local population equates or is close to (at 2 points above or below) the national average in 9 Regions (Yorkshire, NE Thames, SE Thames, Wessex, Oxford, Mersey, N. Western, Wales and N. Ireland); is well above the

110

average in Trent and SW Thames, and markedly so in East Anglia and S. Western; but is well below the average in NW Thames and markedly so in Northern, W. Midlands and Scotland. Special HA is of course omitted from this analysis because it has no local population.

27. It is possible to add to these figures the 1,669 total LASS WTEs, and for the UK as a whole, after adjustment for nonresponse, this provides an estimated overall ratio of 0.27 WTEs per 1,000 population. An important question is whether LASS posts commonly compensate for NHS deficiencies in Regions (or specific District/ Areas) but because of the variable response rates in the survey, and the general lack of correspondence between NHS and LASS administrative areas within individual Health Regions, this cannot be easily answered. In the Northern Region, however, the respective administrative areas happen to be coterminous and there was furthermore a 100% response rate from OT Departments in both the NHS and the LASS. Yet estimates of the effect of adding the LASS to NHS posts showed that Northern's overall OT WTEs/1,000 population ratio remained below the national average which would seem to suggest that no systematic attempt has so far been made within this Region at least to use LASS resources as a means of compensating for NHS deficiencies.

Numbers and distribution of unfilled WTEs

(a) national totals for both the NHS and the LASSs

28. Table 3 shows that for all categories of NHS OT staff throughout the country, 96 WTEs, 0.84% of all WTEs established, had been permanently cut during the period under review; 128.9, or 1.1% had been temporarily frozen

either because of lack of resources or because they had remained unfilled; and 1,149.6, or 10% were designated as vacant as at 31.3.88. In other words, there was an overall total of unfilled 1,374.8 WTEs in the NHS OT Departments surveyed.

29. Equivalent figures for LASS staff show a fairly close correspondence with NHS percentages for unfilled posts. As at 31.3.88: 2 WTEs, 0.12% of all WTEs established, had been permanently cut since 1.4.87; 23 WTEs, 1.4%, had been frozen; and 196 WTEs, 11.8%, were vacant. This gives an overall total of 221 unfilled WTEs in the 86 LASS, surveyed as at 31.3.88.

(b) regional distribution of unfilled NHS WTEs

30. Stating the NHS situation in regional terms: Table 1, already referred to, shows that in 6 of the Regions over 90% of the established WTEs surveyed were filled and that in 11 Regions between 83-89% were filled; in Special HA, by contrast, only 76.9% of the established WTEs were filled.

31. As far as the relatively small numbers of cut or frozen WTEs are concerned, it can be noted from Table 1 that, with the exception of the Special HA, there were instances of some WTEs being cut or frozen in all Regions. The number of cuts range from a high of 20 WTEs in S. Western and 14 in N. Western to 2 in East Anglia, 1 in N. Ireland and 0.4 in Scotland, with Yorkshire and Mersey and Special HA registering no cuts. The number of frozen WTEs ranges from 25 in Scotland, 13 in N. Western and 11 in W. Midlands to 1.5 in NW Thames, 1 in NE Thames and 0.4 in East Anglia.

However, the significance of these numbers obviously relates both to the percentage which they represent of all established WTEs in the particular Region and of course to the much larger number and percentage of the vacant posts.

32. The unavoidable relativity of the statistics involved, and therefore the complexity of the task of drawing accurate inferences from comparative regional data, can be briefly illustrated by analysing parallel figures for a single pair of regions juxtaposed in Table 1. Northern and Yorkshire, for example, happen to show total numbers for cut, frozen and vacant WTEs of 78 and 80 respectively. But because Northern had an established complement of only 508 WTEs at the beginning of the year period compared with Yorkshire's 823, its unfilled WTEs represented almost twice as high a percentage of its OT work force. The possible practical implications of this differential are further highlighted when these percentages are set against the respective overall distributions of established NHS OT WTEs per 1,000 population in Table 2, where it is shown that Northern had a distribution of 0.16 established and 0.14 filled WTEs compared with Yorkshire's figures of 0.23 and 0.20.

Distribution of vacant NHS WTEs

33. An analysis of the figures in the last column of Table 3 indicates that there are major differentials in the vacancy rates as between the various staff categories, especially in respect to the qualified posts. Thus only 7 of the 169 established District WTEs, or 4.1%, were vacant as at 31.3.88 compared with: 112, or 9.6% of the 1,167 Head WTEs; 490, 14.1% of the 3,479 Senior WTEs; and 412, or 25.4% of the 1,623 Basic WTEs.

34. Although, as might be expected, the largest number of these vacancies occurred in the Senior category with the largest number of establishments, it is worth observing that the percentage of vacant Basic WTEs was nearly twice that for Senior WTEs. Indeed it was found that while this key Basic category, where newly qualified recruits normally enter the profession, contained only 25.2% of all qualified posts it also accounted for about 40.2% of the total number of vacancies for all qualified OTs. Lastly it can be noted that in the overall category of qualified staff, vacant WTEs at 31.3.88 totalled 1,022 or 15.9% of the 6,439 established WTEs. In contrast, among all categories of unqualified staff there were only 128 vacant WTEs, representing 2.6% of the total number of the 4,987 WTEs established.

35. Turning to consider the regional distribution of vacant WTEs shown in the last column of Table 1, it can be seen that the variations were extensive. Vacant WTEs numbered well over 100 in as many as 4 Regions: Trent (with an established WTEs/1,000 population ratio of 0.25), NE Thames (ratio 0.24), SE Thames (ratio 0.23) and W. Midlands (ratio 0.18); while SW Thames (ratio 0.25) had 99.7 vacant WTEs. In the middle range there were 6 Regions with vacant WTEs numbering between 55-71: Northern, Yorkshire, NW Thames, Wessex, S. Western, Wales. Except for Special HA, the remaining Regions had vacant WTEs numbering from 32 in N. Ireland and Scotland to 45 in N. Western.

36. There are also considerable regional differentials in the vacancy rates for each NHS OT staff category. This particularly applies to the qualified posts. For example, the vacancy rate for the Basic category ranged from a low of 14.7 and 15.7% in East Anglia and Oxford to a high of

43.9 and 35.8% in SE Thames and Northern. Less dramatically, the rate for Seniors extends from 7.6% in N. Western to 25.5% in Wales. There would appear to be no readily discernible geographic pattern underlying the regional distribution of these kinds of differentials.

Number of weeks WTEs remained unfilled

37. Table 4 shows the number of weeks unfilled WTEs at 31.3.88 had remained respectively cut, frozen or vacant both for qualified and unqualified NHS staff and few LASS staff. About 60% of NHS WTEs for qualified OTs and for LASS OTs had been vacant for over 3 months, while this was true for only 40% of the NHS WTEs for unqualified OTs.

38. There were also substantial percentages of posts which had obviously been vacant for a considerable length of time but less than the 3 month period from which the DHSS starts to count a post as being vacant (see paragraph 16 above). Yet any vacancy which continues for more than a couple of weeks is likely to cause serious difficulties for a busy OT Department, particularly if already understaffed; a vacancy certainly does not became a matter of concern only after it has lasted for 12 or more weeks.

Functional allocation of WTEs

(a) in the NHS

39. Table 5 gives the national distribution of established WTEs to the 8 specified functional areas designated in the questionnaire, together with the percentages of

qualified WTEs and of the vacancies for all established WTEs in each area. Although by far the highest number of WTEs were assigned respectively to the Mentally Ill and Geriatric patients, the differential between them was major, with the allocation to the Mentally Ill being over 1,000 more WTEs than to Geriatrics. The next largest number of WTEs was assigned to the Mentally Handicapped. Administration, at 8.8%, accounted for considerably more WTEs than any of the remaining areas while, perhaps rather surprisingly, Paediatrics was at the bottom of the list with a mere 2.8% of the WTEs.

40. It was also instructive to discover that under 50% of all WTEs assigned to the three largest allocations – Mentally Ill, Geriatrics and Mentally Handicapped – were for qualified staff. This is in noticeable contrast to the very high percentages of qualified WTEs devoted (in descending order) respectively to Paediatrics, Community work, Acute Medicine, Administration and Acute Surgery.

41. The national percentage rates of vacant WTEs in the different functional areas are shown to be much less uneven than those for the various staff categories given in Table 3, running at about 8% in 5 of the functional areas, but with higher rates in Acute Medicine, the Mentally Ill and the Mentally Handicapped.

42. Table 6 might provide a useful tool for any subsequent assessment, which could perhaps be undertaken by both COT and the MPAG, of appropriate OT staff-patient ratios in respect of the different client groups, taking the current functional allocation of WTEs within the Regions as a starting point. For the immediate

purposes of the present survey it can be said to reveal disturbingly high levels of differentials in these allocations as between the various Regions. Thus for each of the 7 functional areas directly concerned with patient care (i.e. excluding Administration and 'Other' functions) there are instances where the WTE allocations are seemingly unaccountably much higher or much lower than the overall national percentage given in the second column of Table 5.

43. To cite two of the more striking examples of highest and lowest ratings: S. Western Region allocated 20.9% of its WTE's for the Mentally Handicapped while NW Thames devoted a startlingly low 2.2% to the same group, compared with a national average of 11.4%. For Community work N. Ireland allocated 14.8% while Mersey and Scotland allocated only 1.0%, compared with a national average of 3.6%. The extent to which such differentials can be said to have any genuine equivalence to actual differentials in the number of patients in the respective regional client groups or merely reflect differences of attitudes and policies remains to be determined by further research. But in the case of N. Ireland, for example, one could perhaps make an immediate assumption that the main reason why a comparatively high proportion of WTEs is devoted to Community work must be due to the existing integration of its health and social services, referred to in paragraph 12. Certainly there would seem to be no prima facie grounds for supposing there are more people in need of community care in N. Ireland than in Mersey or Scotland or anywhere else in the United Kingdom.

44. Table 7 relates the WTE allocation for Geriatrics specifically to population statistics for the 75+ age-group.

It shows that for every 1,000 people in the United Kingdom aged 75 and over there were 0.63 established WTEs devoted to Geriatric patients, a ratio which, although it is nearly 3 times the overall national distribution of all established OT WTEs per 1,000 population, nevertheless bears little relationship to the relative needs of the elderly. The regional differentials are once again striking, with many of the ratings either much higher or much lower than the national average. To take the case of the two Regions showing respectively the highest and lowest rating: N. Ireland has an allocation of 0.92 WTEs for Geriatrics per 1,000 population aged 75+, which is 0.29 more than the national figure; while NW Thames has an allocation of 0.39, which is 0.24 below the national figure. With respect to the distribution of WTEs for qualified staff, N. Ireland heads the list with a ratio of 0.49, while NW Thames is at the bottom of the scale with 0.23. Taking only the filled WTEs for qualified OTs, N. Ireland remains at the top with a distribution of 0.41, although NW Thames has been replaced in bottom position by SE Thames with 0.16 distribution.

(b) in the LASSs

45. There are no corresponding figures for the LASSs, which categorise care groups in a different way, but Table 8 shows that almost half the WTEs were allocated to Adult Physical Handicap. Unfortunately there was no separate classification in the questionnaire for a WTE allocation specifically to care for the elderly.

Reasons for staff leaving posts

46. During the year period surveyed 1,217 NHS staff left their posts. Most of them, however, remained in the

profession: 915 merely changed their posts within the NHS (558 were promoted, 319 moved to other posts in the same grade, and 38 were demoted), but 189 moved out of the NHS – 113 to go to Local Authority employment, 48 to emigrate and 28 to return to their home country.

47. Table 9 shows a total of 549 NHS staff leaving the profession, which represents approximately 4% of all established posts included in the survey. The largest number left for domestic reasons: 102 to become mothers, and 75 because of other family commitments – more than half of this group came from the Senior category of qualified staff. The next largest number, 131, chose to take up another career and the majority of these personnel were unqualified staff. Sixty-nine personnel retired, the majority of them unqualified staff. Most of the remaining 172 departed the profession for reasons specified as 'holiday/ travel', 'study', 'unemployed', and 'ill-health', but 44 left for 'other' reasons. There were also movements out of OT in the LASS posts, the largest proportion, 31 out of 98, being because of pregnancy.

48. It should be appreciated that the categories of reasons for staff leaving posts and/or the profession which were specified respectively in footnotes * and footnote ** to the questionnaires are not entirely satisfactory. For example, no provision is made under footnote * to indicate OTs intending to enter private practice, and the fact that a number of them emigrated or returned to their home country cannot be taken as convincing evidence of an intention to stay in the profession; nor, under footnote ** is the desire to take a 'holiday' or to 'study' clear evidence of their leaving it. Due to the looseness of the definitions in this part of the

questionnaire, the numbers of 549 NHS and 98 LASS staff leaving the profession should not necessarily be assumed accurately to reflect the true situation.

Intake and sources of new recruits

49. Approximately 8% of all established NHS posts were filled by new recruits during the year period. But Table 9 shows that by far the largest numbers of these in fact came from other posts within the NHS and therefore should probably be assumed to have been already included in the 915 staff referred to in paragraph 46 as having 'changed' their NHS posts. Nevertheless the table also shows an intake of 372 newly qualified OTs into the Basic category and an overall intake of 428 recruits *excluding* those from other NHS posts. The intake into the Senior category excluding recruits from within the NHS was 238, but they came precisely from other NHS posts, most of them almost certainly having been promoted from the Basic category. It should be noted too that 92 of the 139 staff re-entering the NHS after a 'break' also went into the Senior category. In the Helper category there was an intake of 251 recruits to established posts excluding those from within the NHS but including 197 from unspecified 'Other' sources. In the LASSs the largest number of new recruits, 130 out of 303, re-entered after a 'break'; only 22 came from the NHS, while relatively larger numbers moved from the LASSs to the NHS, 79 out of the 1,094 new entrants.

50. Overall, it appears that in the year surveyed movements into the profession were approximately twice the number of movements out, and many of the latter were from the qualified posts.

Concluding observations

51. The summary of key statistics which follows these concluding remarks lists the more significant of the national totals relating to current OT staffing levels both in the NHS and the LASSs. Unfortunately there is no effective means of similarly extracting the very important and illuminating differentials in the regional totals or in the allocation of WTEs to individual clinical functional areas, except by referring directly to the tables (Nos 1, 2, 5, 6 and 7). It is also partly for this reason that considerable emphasis has been given to illustrating such differentials in the paper (paragraphs 25-26, 31-32, 35-36, 39, 42-44).

52. The overarching issue to be considered when trying to assess the implications of the distributions of national OT staffing levels must surely turn on the question of whether the basic ratio of 0.27 total established WTEs per 1,000 population can be regarded as adequate to meet the real needs of patients, taking into account the expanding group of people aged over 75, the substantial portion of established WTEs that may happen to be unfilled at any given time and the fact that several Health Regions in any case have a WTE/population ratio well below the national average. These considerations can only reinforce existing concern about the high and regionally variable proportion of posts for qualified OTs that have remained vacant for long periods of time, the high rate of movements in and out of the profession and the general problem of recruitment to both NHS and LASS Departments.

53. A new and detailed assessment of the appropriate OT/patient ratios required to meet the needs of all the

different types of client groups should be undertaken as a matter of priority in order to provide a basis for rational future planning and effective matching of OT supply and demand. It is hoped that the comprehensive set of data gathered in this survey can make a useful contribution towards achieving that objective.

Summary of key statistics, national totals applicable at 31.3.88

(Figures refer only to OT Departments included in the survey, based on a 91% response rate to the NHS questionnaire and a 74% response rate to the LASS questionnaire)

		Initial Paragraph Reference	*Table Nos*
(i) Total Established Posts/WTEs			
NHS	13,615/11,426.1	22	3
LASS	31,992/1,669.2	23	
(ii) Qualified/Unqualified			
NHS Established WTEs	6,439.9/4,987.1	24	
(iii) Unfilled WTEs			
NHS	1,374.8	28	3
LASS	221	29	
(iv) WTEs Designated Vacant			3
NHS Qual/Unqual	1,022/128	34	
LASS	196	29	
(v) WTEs Vacant 31.3.88 for more than 12 weeks			
NHS Qual/Unqual	648/42		4
LASS	108		4
(vi) Staff Leaving the Profession			
from NHS	549	47	8
from LASS	98	47	

1987-8 Staffing Levels for OT Departments

		Initial Paragraph Reference	*Table Nos*
(vii) Intake of Newly Qualified Recruits			
to NHS posts	411		
to LASS posts	23		
(viii) Total Established WTEs			
per 1,000 UK Population	0.27	27	
(ix) NHS Established WTEs per		26	2
1,000 UK Population			
Established	0.22		
Filled	0.19		
Established Qual/Unqual	0.12/0.10		
Filled Qual/Unqual	0.10/0.09		
(x) NHS Established WTEs allocated		44	7
to Geriatrics per 1,000			
Population aged 75+			
Established Qual/Unqual	0.31/0.32		
Filled Qual/Unqual	0.30/0.31		

Table 1. Regional distribution of established NHS WTEs included in survey

Region		WTEs at 31.3.88				Total
		Filled	Cut	Frozen	Vacant	
Northern	No.	429.7	10	11	57.0	507.7
	%	84.6	2.0	2.1	11.2	100.0
Yorkshire	No.	750.3	0	8.5	71.2	830.0
	%	90.4	0	1.0	8.6	100.0
Trent	No.	797.3	3	8.7	111.8	920.8
	%	86.6	0.3	0.9	12.1	100.0
East Anglia	No.	442.1	2	0.4	38.6	483.1
	%	91.5	0.4	0.1	8.0	100.0
NW Thames	No.	420.2	3	1.5	68.1	492.8
	%	85.3	0.6	0.3	13.8	100.0
NE Thames	No.	757.4	3.9	1	114.6	876.9
	%	86.4	0.4	0.1	13.1	100.0
SE Thames	No.	618.2	3	5.9	119.1	746.2
	%	82.8	0.4	0.8	16.0	100.0
SW Thames	No.	567.2	8.8	9.5	99.7	685.2
	%	82.8	1.3	1.4	14.5	100.0
Wessex	No.	599.4	4.2	3.8	55.8	663.2
	%	90.4	0.6	0.6	8.4	100.0
Oxford	No.	473.4	2.3	2.1	36.4	514.2
	%	92.1	0.4	0.4	7.1	100.0
South Western	No.	780.7	20.1	6.1	56.9	863.7
	%	90.4	2.3	0.7	6.6	100.0
West Midlands	No.	784.9	8	10.7	100.0	904.6
	%	86.8	0.9	1.2	11.1	100.0
Mersey	No.	443.4	0	10.0	40.5	493.9
	%	89.8	0	2.0	8.2	100.0
North Western	No.	638.7	13.7	13.1	44.9	710.4
	%	89.9	1.9	1.9	6.3	100.0
Wales	No.	430.2	12.9	8.6	57.2	508.9
	%	84.5	2.5	1.7	11.3	100.0
Northern Ireland	No.	281.0	1	3.0	31.6	316.6
	%	88.8	0.3	0.9	10.0	100.0
Special HA	No.	44.5	0	0	13.3	57.8
	%	76.9	0	0	23.1	100.0
Scotland	No.	792.5	0.4	25.2	31.9	850.0
	%	93.2	0.1	2.9	3.9	100.0
TOTAL	No.	10051.3	96.3	128.9	1149.6	11426.1
	%	88.0	0.8	1.1	10.1	100.0

Table 2. Regional distribution of qualified and unqualified NHS WTEs per 1,000 population at 31.3.88

Region	Established WTEs			Filled WTEs		
	Qual.	Unqual.	All	Qual.	Unqual.	All
Northern	0.09	0.07	0.16	0.07	0.07	0.14
Yorkshire	0.10	0.13	0.23	0.08	0.12	0.20
Trent	0.15	0.10	0.25	0.12	0.09	0.21
East Anglia	0.16	0.11	0.27	0.14	0.11	0.25
NW Thames	0.13	0.06	0.19	0.10	0.05	0.15
NE Thames	0.12	0.12	0.24	0.09	0.12	0.21
SE Thames	0.12	0.11	0.23	0.09	0.10	0.19
SW Thames	0.14	0.11	0.25	0.11	0.10	0.21
Wessex	0.13	0.10	0.23	0.11	0.10	0.21
Oxford	0.13	0.07	0.20	0.12	0.07	0.19
S Western	0.15	0.14	0.29	0.13	0.13	0.26
W Midlands	0.10	0.08	0.18	0.08	0.07	0.15
Mersey	0.12	0.08	0.20	0.10	0.08	0.18
N Western	0.12	0.10	0.22	0.10	0.09	0.19
Wales	0.12	0.12	0.24	0.09	0.11	0.20
N Ireland	0.14	0.07	0.21	0.12	0.06	0.18
Scotland	0.11	0.07	0.18	0.10	0.07	0.17
TOTAL*	0.12	0.10	0.22	0.10	0.09	0.19

Adjustment made for non-response - population estimates taken from Population Trends 53 (OPCS) for 1987.

* Including Special HA.

Table 3. Filled and unfilled NHS WTEs per staff category, national totals at 31.3.88

Category		WTEs				
		Filled	Cut	Frozen	Vacant	Total
District	No	161.1	0.0	1.0	7.0	169.1
	%	95.27	0.00	0.59	4.14	1.5
Head	No	1033.3	12.0	10.0	112.0	1167.3
	%	88.52	1.03	0.86	9.59	10.2
Senior	No	2921.4	25.4	42.5	489.8	3479.2
	%	83.97	0.73	1.22	14.08	30.4
Basic	No	1160.6	23.0	27.5	412.3	1623.4
	%	71.49	1.42	1.69	25.40	14.2
Helper TI	No	1347.2	3.0	24.3	32.2	1406.7
	%	95.77	0.21	1.73	2.29	12.3
Helper	No	2327.4	26.3	17.1	67.1	2437.8
	%	95.47	1.08	0.70	2.75	21.3
TI	No	696.7	5.5	4.7	17.9	724.8
	%	96.12	0.76	0.65	2.47	6.3
Therap	No	159.4	1.0	0.0	2.5	162.9
	%	97.80	0.63	0.00	1.57	1.4
Other	No	244.3	0.0	1.9	8.7	254.9
	%	95.84	0.00	0.74	3.42	2.2
TOTAL	No	10051.3	96.3	128.9	1149.6	11426.1
	%	88.0	0.84	1.1	10.0	100.0

126

Table 4. Number of weeks WTEs remained unfilled, unqualified and qualified NHS + LASS staff

Weeks Unfilled		NHS WTEs							
		Cut		Frozen		Vacant		All Unfilled	
		Qual.	Unqual.	Qual.	Unqual.	Qual.	Unqual.	Qual.	Unqual.
Under 7	No	17	13	17	11	189	33	223	57
	%	29.8	36.1	20.7	22.4	18.5	25.8	19.2	26.8
7-12	No	2	1	9	5	108	29	119	35
	%	3.5	2.8	11.0	10.5	10.6	22.7	10.2	16.4
More than 12	No	30	12	49	30	648	42	727	84
	%	52.6	33.3	59.8	61.2	63.4	32.8	62.8	39.4
Not known	No	8	10	7	3	77	24	92	37
	%	14.0	27.8	8.5	6.1	7.5	18.8	7.9	17.4
Total	No	57	36	82	49	1022	128	1161	213
	%	100	100	100	100	100	100	100	100

Weeks Unfilled		LASS WTEs			
		Cut	Frozen	Vacant	All Unfilled
Under 7	No	0	1	20	21
	%	0	4.3	10.2	9.5
7-12	No	0	2	36	38
	%	0	8.7	18.4	17.2
More than 12	No	2	18	108	128
	%	100	78.3	55.1	57.9
Not known	No	0	2	32	34
	%	0	8.7	16.3	15.4
Total	No	2	23	196	221
	%	100	100	100	100

127

Table 5. Functional allocation of NHS WTEs, national totals

Functional Designation	Established WTEs Allocated	% of all Established WTEs	% of WTEs Allocation Qualified	% of WTES Allocation Vacant at 31.3.88
Acute Medicine	760.2	6.7	74.0	9.6
Acute Surgery	554.7	4.9	73.5	8.5
Geriatrics	2365.0	20.7	49.8	8.7
Paediatrics	323.0	2.8	87.2	8.7
Community	415.7	3.6	82.6	8.4
Mentally Ill	3624.5	31.7	49.9	10.5
Mental Handicap	1298.8	11.4	40.8	12.3
Administration	999.9	8.8	73.9	8.7
Total (incl. 'Other' Functions)	11426.1	100.0	56.4	10.0

Table 6. Functional allocation of NHS established WTEs* in different regions as at 31.3.88

		Geriat.	Ment. Hand.	Acute Med.	Acute Surg.	Paed.	Comm.	Ment. Ill	Admin.	Other	Total
Northern	No	121	31	29	14	8	16	158	60		508
	%	23.8	6.1	5.7	2.8	1.6	3.1	31.1	11.8	14.8	100
Yorkshire	No	172	144	58	38	18	15	269	74		830
	%	20.7	17.3	7.0	4.6	2.2	1.8	32.4	8.9	5.1	100
Trent	No	175	110	54	30	27	21	298	58		921
	%	19.0	11.9	5.9	3.3	2.9	2.3	32.4	6.3	16.0	100
E Anglia	No	100	65	18	16	18	15	127	23		483
	%	20.7	13.5	3.7	3.3	3.7	3.1	26.3	4.8	20.9	100
NW Thames	No	85	11	52	38	19	27	171	43		493
	%	17.2	2.2	10.5	9.7	3.9	5.5	34.7	8.7	9.6	100
NE Thames	No	158	110	85	53	24	14	300	92		877
	%	18.0	12.5	9.7	6.0	2.7	1.6	34.2	10.2	4.8	100
SE Thames	No	142	88	58	35	22	16	257	63		746
	%	19.0	11.8	7.8	4.7	2.9	2.1	34.5	8.4	9.8	100
SW Thames	No	120	121	40	40	16	12	231	66		685
	%	17.5	17.7	5.8	5.8	2.3	1.8	33.7	9.6	5.8	100
Wessex	No	141	59	42	35	23	17	202	53		663
	%	21.3	8.9	5.3	5.3	3.5	2.6	30.5	8.0	13.6	100
Oxford	No	102	53	25	19	11	73	115	41		514
	%	19.8	10.3	4.9	3.7	2.1	14.2	22.4	8.0	14.6	100
S Western	No	188	181	59	38	9	14	258	61		864
	%	21.8	20.9	6.8	4.4	1.0	1.6	29.9	7.1	6.5	100
W Mids.	No	204	90	64	70	20	51	260	68		904
	%	22.5	9.9	7.1	7.7	2.2	5.6	28.7	7.5	8.8	100
Mersey	No	104	60	39	24	18	4	163	47		494
	%	21.1	12.1	7.9	4.9	3.6	1.0	33.0	9.5	6.9	100
N West.	No	160	20	43	45	27	41	252	69		710
	%	22.5	2.8	6.1	6.3	3.8	5.8	35.5	9.7	9.5	100
Wales	No	115	49	22	16	7	27	197	37		509
	%	22.6	9.6	4.3	3.1	1.4	5.3	38.7	7.3	8.0	100
N Ireland	No	71	22	20	15	13	47	77	30		316
	%	22.4	6.9	6.3	4.7	4.1	14.8	24.3	9.5	7.0	100
Scotland	No	207	81	54	29	41	6	256	108		851
	%	24.3	9.5	6.3	3.4	4.8	1.0	31.3	12.7	6.7	100
Spec. HA	No	–	2	1	–	–	1	25	8		58
	%		3.4	1.7			1.7	43.1	13.8	36.3	100
Total	No	2365	1299	760	555	823	416	3624	1000		11426
	%	20.7	11.4	6.7	4.9	2.8	3.6	31.7	8.8	9.4	100

* rounded up

Table 7. Regional distribution of NHS WTEs allocated to geriatrics per 1,000 population* aged 75+ as at 31.3.88

	Established WTEs			Filled WTEs		
	Qualified	Unqualified	All	Qualified	Unqualified	All
Northern	0.26	0.36	0.62	0.21	0.36	0.57
Yorkshire	0.31	0.40	0.71	0.25	0.38	0.63
Trent	0.37	0.22	0.59	0.32	0.21	0.52
East Anglia	0.39	0.31	0.70	0.32	0.31	0.32
NW Thames	0.23	0.16	0.39	0.20	0.16	0.36
NE Thames	0.28	0.35	0.62	0.20	0.33	0.53
SE Thames	0.24	0.26	0.50	0.16	0.26	0.41
SW Thames	0.32	0.21	0.53	0.25	0.19	0.44
Wessex	0.30	0.33	0.63	0.28	0.32	0.60
Oxford	0.36	0.40	0.76	0.31	0.39	0.70
S.Western	0.31	0.42	0.73	0.27	0.42	0.69
W. Midlands	0.33	0.33	0.66	0.25	0.33	0.57
Mersey	0.38	0.31	0.69	0.31	0.31	0.62
N.Western	0.27	0.33	0.60	0.23	0.25	0.55
Wales	0.31	0.28	0.59	0.31	0.41	0.82
N.Ireland	0.49	0.43	0.92	0.41	0.32	0.63
Scotland	0.33	0.32	0.65	0.31	0.32	0.63
Total **	0.31	0.32	0.63	0.26	0.31	0.57

*   Not corrected for missing Districts
** Including Special HA

Table 8. Functional allocation of LASS WTEs, national totals

Functional Area/ Designation	WTEs Allocated	% of all WTEs Established
Adult Phys. Handicap	778.8	46.7
Mental Health	11.5	0.7
Mental Handicap	16.1	1.0
Children	44.6	2.7
Day Care	32.6	2.3
Residential Care	25.5	1.5
Housing	17.9	1.1
Management	168.8	10.1
Other	573.8	34.4

Table 9. Categorisation of movements in and out of occupational therapy 1.4.87 – 31.3.88, NHS and LASS

Movements Out	From NHS Posts										From LASS Posts
	Dist.	Head	Sen.	Bas.	Help. TI	Help.	TI	Ther.	Oth.	All NHS	
Another career	3	2	19	6	22	59	10	2	8	131	16
Holiday	0	4	22	6	0	7	0	0	0	39	4
Study	0	2	10	1	4	8	0	0	1	26	1
Unemployed	0	2	12	2	3	11	0	0	1	31	7
Maternity	1	17	56	11	5	7	1	3	1	102	31
Domestic	1	6	29	3	6	27	1	0	2	75	14
Ill-health	0	0	5	3	6	15	3	0	0	32	7
Retirement	2	5	6	2	12	26	12	0	4	69	12
Other	0	0	5	4	9	21	3	0	2	44	6
Total	7	38	164	38	67	181	30	5	19	549	98

New Recruits	To NHS Posts										To LASS Posts
Newly qualified	0	3	20	372	4	2	3	6	1	411	23
Further training	1	8	32	6	2	3	2	1	0	55	13
LASS	1	11	37	3	5	13	6	2	1	79	72
Break	0	8	92	26	1	10	1	0	1	139	130
Private practice	0	2	6	0	0	0	2	0	1	11	34
Abroad	0	3	27	18	2	26	2	0	2	80	3
Other	1	3	24	3	44	197	21	3	23	319	6
Other NHS posts*	10	122	478	96	25	51	17	5	8	812	22
Total excl. NHS posts	3	38	238	428	58	251	37	12	29	1094	303
Total in Survey	173	1213	4149	1787	1689	3225	799	217	398	3615	1922

* See text on new recruits

Annexes

Annexe 1 (a) Sample page from NHS questionnaire

Page No. |0 | 2|

Post No	Title of Post	Enter Grade	Date Post Created			No. of Hours per week 36=FT	No. of weeks vacant or 00=filled	If post vacant now tick as appropriate			
			Before 1.4.87	Since 1.4.87	After 1.4.88			Perm./ Cut	Frozen/ No resources	Frozen because unfilled	Funded No recruit
0 0	Example										
0 1	Head										
0 2	Head										
0 3	Head										
0 4	Head										
0 5	Head										
0 6	Head										
0 7	Head										
0 8	Head										
0 9	Head										
1 0	Head										
1 1	Head										
1 2	Head										
1 3	Head										
1 4	Head										
1 5	Head										
1 6	Head										
1 7	Head										
1 8	Head										
1 9	Head										
2 0	Head										
2 1	Head										
2 2	Head										
2 3	Head										
2 4	Head										
2 5	Head										
2 6	Head										
2 7	Head										
2 8	Head										
2 9	Head										

*   Moved in OT: a = same grade;   b = promotion;   c = lower grade;   d = local authority;
** Moved out OT: a = another career; b = holiday/travel; c = study;   d = unemployed;
+   New recruit: a = newly qualified; b = further training; c = from NHS post; d = from LA post;

Hours established/week whether filled or not: **MUST EQUAL TOTAL HOURS** (enter no. hours or leave blank as approp.) **ESTABLISHED**									Tick if Clinical Supervis Allowance received	If postholder changed since 1.4.87 enter codes as below		
Ac. Med	Ac. Surg	Ger- iat.	Paed- iat.	Comm- unity	Ment- ill.	Ment- Hand.	Admin.	Other		Left post - _either_ stayed : gone out in OT* : of OT**		New+ recruit from
⊔ ⊔	⊔ ⊔	⊔ ⊔	⊔ ⊔	⊔ ⊔	⊔ ⊔	⊔ ⊔	⊔ ⊔	⊔ ⊔	—	: —	: —	—
⊔ ⊔	⊔ ⊔	⊔ ⊔	⊔ ⊔	⊔ ⊔	⊔ ⊔	⊔ ⊔	⊔ ⊔	⊔ ⊔	—	: —	: —	—
⊔ ⊔	⊔ ⊔	⊔ ⊔	⊔ ⊔	⊔ ⊔	⊔ ⊔	⊔ ⊔	⊔ ⊔	⊔ ⊔	—	: —	: —	—
⊔ ⊔	⊔ ⊔	⊔ ⊔	⊔ ⊔	⊔ ⊔	⊔ ⊔	⊔ ⊔	⊔ ⊔	⊔ ⊔	—	: —	: —	—
⊔ ⊔	⊔ ⊔	⊔ ⊔	⊔ ⊔	⊔ ⊔	⊔ ⊔	⊔ ⊔	⊔ ⊔	⊔ ⊔	—	: —	: —	—
⊔ ⊔	⊔ ⊔	⊔ ⊔	⊔ ⊔	⊔ ⊔	⊔ ⊔	⊔ ⊔	⊔ ⊔	⊔ ⊔	—	: —	: —	—
⊔ ⊔	⊔ ⊔	⊔ ⊔	⊔ ⊔	⊔ ⊔	⊔ ⊔	⊔ ⊔	⊔ ⊔	⊔ ⊔	—	: —	: —	—
⊔ ⊔	⊔ ⊔	⊔ ⊔	⊔ ⊔	⊔ ⊔	⊔ ⊔	⊔ ⊔	⊔ ⊔	⊔ ⊔	—	: —	: —	—
⊔ ⊔	⊔ ⊔	⊔ ⊔	⊔ ⊔	⊔ ⊔	⊔ ⊔	⊔ ⊔	⊔ ⊔	⊔ ⊔	—	: —	: —	—
⊔ ⊔	⊔ ⊔	⊔ ⊔	⊔ ⊔	⊔ ⊔	⊔ ⊔	⊔ ⊔	⊔ ⊔	⊔ ⊔	—	: —	: —	—
⊔ ⊔	⊔ ⊔	⊔ ⊔	⊔ ⊔	⊔ ⊔	⊔ ⊔	⊔ ⊔	⊔ ⊔	⊔ ⊔	—	: —	: —	—
⊔ ⊔	⊔ ⊔	⊔ ⊔	⊔ ⊔	⊔ ⊔	⊔ ⊔	⊔ ⊔	⊔ ⊔	⊔ ⊔	—	: —	: —	—
⊔ ⊔	⊔ ⊔	⊔ ⊔	⊔ ⊔	⊔ ⊔	⊔ ⊔	⊔ ⊔	⊔ ⊔	⊔ ⊔	—	: —	: —	—
⊔ ⊔	⊔ ⊔	⊔ ⊔	⊔ ⊔	⊔ ⊔	⊔ ⊔	⊔ ⊔	⊔ ⊔	⊔ ⊔	—	: —	: —	—
⊔ ⊔	⊔ ⊔	⊔ ⊔	⊔ ⊔	⊔ ⊔	⊔ ⊔	⊔ ⊔	⊔ ⊔	⊔ ⊔	—	: —	: —	—
⊔ ⊔	⊔ ⊔	⊔ ⊔	⊔ ⊔	⊔ ⊔	⊔ ⊔	⊔ ⊔	⊔ ⊔	⊔ ⊔	—	: —	: —	—
⊔ ⊔	⊔ ⊔	⊔ ⊔	⊔ ⊔	⊔ ⊔	⊔ ⊔	⊔ ⊔	⊔ ⊔	⊔ ⊔	—	: —	: —	—
⊔ ⊔	⊔ ⊔	⊔ ⊔	⊔ ⊔	⊔ ⊔	⊔ ⊔	⊔ ⊔	⊔ ⊔	⊔ ⊔	—	: —	: —	—
⊔ ⊔	⊔ ⊔	⊔ ⊔	⊔ ⊔	⊔ ⊔	⊔ ⊔	⊔ ⊔	⊔ ⊔	⊔ ⊔	—	: —	: —	—
⊔ ⊔	⊔ ⊔	⊔ ⊔	⊔ ⊔	⊔ ⊔	⊔ ⊔	⊔ ⊔	⊔ ⊔	⊔ ⊔	—	: —	: —	—
⊔ ⊔	⊔ ⊔	⊔ ⊔	⊔ ⊔	⊔ ⊔	⊔ ⊔	⊔ ⊔	⊔ ⊔	⊔ ⊔	—	: —	: —	—
⊔ ⊔	⊔ ⊔	⊔ ⊔	⊔ ⊔	⊔ ⊔	⊔ ⊔	⊔ ⊔	⊔ ⊔	⊔ ⊔	—	: —	: —	—
⊔ ⊔	⊔ ⊔	⊔ ⊔	⊔ ⊔	⊔ ⊔	⊔ ⊔	⊔ ⊔	⊔ ⊔	⊔ ⊔	—	: —	: —	—
⊔ ⊔	⊔ ⊔	⊔ ⊔	⊔ ⊔	⊔ ⊔	⊔ ⊔	⊔ ⊔	⊔ ⊔	⊔ ⊔	—	: —	: —	—
⊔ ⊔	⊔ ⊔	⊔ ⊔	⊔ ⊔	⊔ ⊔	⊔ ⊔	⊔ ⊔	⊔ ⊔	⊔ ⊔	—	: —	: —	—

e = return to home country; f = work abroad;   g = other.
e = maternity;   f = other domestic commitment; g = ill-health; h = retirement; i = other.

e = from break;   f = from private practice;   g = from abroad; h = other.

Annexe 1 (b) Sample page from LASS questionnaire

Page No. | 0 | | Based on Funded Establishment as at 31.3.88

Post No	Title of Post	Enter Grade	Date Post Created			No. of Hours per week 36=FT	No. of weeks vacant or 00=filled	If post vacant now tick as appropriate			
			Before 1.4.87	Since 1.4.87	After 1.4.88			Perm./ Cut	Frozen/ No resources	Frozen because unfilled	Funded No recruit
0 0	Rehab. Officer	P01	__ :	__ :	__			__ :	__ :	__ :	__ :
0 1			__ :	__ :	__			__ :	__ :	__ :	__ :
0 2			__ :	__ :	__			__ :	__ :	__ :	__ :
0 3			__ :	__ :	__			__ :	__ :	__ :	__ :
0 4			__ :	__ :	__			__ :	__ :	__ :	__ :
0 5			__ :	__ :	__			__ :	__ :	__ :	__ :
0 6			__ :	__ :	__			__ :	__ :	__ :	__ :
0 7			__ :	__ :	__			__ :	__ :	__ :	__ :
0 8			__ :	__ :	__			__ :	__ :	__ :	__ :
0 9			__ :	__ :	__			__ :	__ :	__ :	__ :
1 0			__ :	__ :	__			__ :	__ :	__ :	__ :
1 1			__ :	__ :	__			__ :	__ :	__ :	__ :
1 2			__ :	__ :	__			__ :	__ :	__ :	__ :
1 3			__ :	__ :	__			__ :	__ :	__ :	__ :
1 4			__ :	__ :	__			__ :	__ :	__ :	__ :
1 5			__ :	__ :	__			__ :	__ :	__ :	__ :
1 6			__ :	__ :	__			__ :	__ :	__ :	__ :
1 7			__ :	__ :	__			__ :	__ :	__ :	__ :
1 8			__ :	__ :	__			__ :	__ :	__ :	__ :
1 9			__ :	__ :	__			__ :	__ :	__ :	__ :
2 0			__ :	__ :	__			__ :	__ :	__ :	__ :
2 1			__ :	__ :	__			__ :	__ :	__ :	__ :
2 2			__ :	__ :	__			__ :	__ :	__ :	__ :
2 3			__ :	__ :	__			__ :	__ :	__ :	__ :
2 4			__ :	__ :	__			__ :	__ :	__ :	__ :
2 5			__ :	__ :	__			__ :	__ :	__ :	__ :
2 6			__ :	__ :	__			__ :	__ :	__ :	__ :
2 7			__ :	__ :	__			__ :	__ :	__ :	__ :
2 8			__ :	__ :	__			__ :	__ :	__ :	__ :
2 9			__ :	__ :	__			__ :	__ :	__ :	__ :

IF POSTHOLDER LEFT, COMPLETE EITHER MOVED IN OR MOVED OUT COLUMN
* Moved in OT: a = same grade;   b = promotion;   c = lower grade;   d = to NHS;
** Moved out OT: a = another career;   b = holiday/travel;   c = study;   d = unemployed;

IF JOB NEWLY FILLED COMPLETE NEW RECRUIT COLUMN - LEAVE BLANK IF JOB NOT FILLED
\+ New recruit: a = newly qualified; b = further training; c = from another LA post; d = from NHS;

Local Authority: No. as on front page | | | | | LA Name: _____

Hours established/week whether filled or not: **MUST EQUAL TOTAL HOURS** (enter no. hours or leave blank as approp.) **ESTABLISHED**									If postholder changed since 1.4.87 enter codes as below	
Adult Phys. Hand.	Mental Health	Mental Hand.	Children	Day Care	Resid. Care	Housing	Manage-ment	Other	Left post - _either_ stayed : gone out in OT° : of OT**	New+ recruit from
|_|	|_|	|_|	|_|	|_|	|_|	|_|	|_|	|_|	__ : __	__
|_|	|_|	|_|	|_|	|_|	|_|	|_|	|_|	|_|	__ : __	__
|_|	|_|	|_|	|_|	|_|	|_|	|_|	|_|	|_|	__ : __	__
|_|	|_|	|_|	|_|	|_|	|_|	|_|	|_|	|_|	__ : __	__
|_|	|_|	|_|	|_|	|_|	|_|	|_|	|_|	|_|	__ : __	__
|_|	|_|	|_|	|_|	|_|	|_|	|_|	|_|	|_|	__ : __	__
|_|	|_|	|_|	|_|	|_|	|_|	|_|	|_|	|_|	__ : __	__
|_|	|_|	|_|	|_|	|_|	|_|	|_|	|_|	|_|	__ : __	__
|_|	|_|	|_|	|_|	|_|	|_|	|_|	|_|	|_|	__ : __	__
|_|	|_|	|_|	|_|	|_|	|_|	|_|	|_|	|_|	__ : __	__
|_|	|_|	|_|	|_|	|_|	|_|	|_|	|_|	|_|	__ : __	__
|_|	|_|	|_|	|_|	|_|	|_|	|_|	|_|	|_|	__ : __	__
|_|	|_|	|_|	|_|	|_|	|_|	|_|	|_|	|_|	__ : __	__
|_|	|_|	|_|	|_|	|_|	|_|	|_|	|_|	|_|	__ : __	__
|_|	|_|	|_|	|_|	|_|	|_|	|_|	|_|	|_|	__ : __	__
|_|	|_|	|_|	|_|	|_|	|_|	|_|	|_|	|_|	__ : __	__
|_|	|_|	|_|	|_|	|_|	|_|	|_|	|_|	|_|	__ : __	__
|_|	|_|	|_|	|_|	|_|	|_|	|_|	|_|	|_|	__ : __	__
|_|	|_|	|_|	|_|	|_|	|_|	|_|	|_|	|_|	__ : __	__
|_|	|_|	|_|	|_|	|_|	|_|	|_|	|_|	|_|	__ : __	__
|_|	|_|	|_|	|_|	|_|	|_|	|_|	|_|	|_|	__ : __	__
|_|	|_|	|_|	|_|	|_|	|_|	|_|	|_|	|_|	__ : __	__
|_|	|_|	|_|	|_|	|_|	|_|	|_|	|_|	|_|	__ : __	__
|_|	|_|	|_|	|_|	|_|	|_|	|_|	|_|	|_|	__ : __	__
|_|	|_|	|_|	|_|	|_|	|_|	|_|	|_|	|_|	__ : __	__
|_|	|_|	|_|	|_|	|_|	|_|	|_|	|_|	|_|	__ : __	__
|_|	|_|	|_|	|_|	|_|	|_|	|_|	|_|	|_|	__ : __	__
|_|	|_|	|_|	|_|	|_|	|_|	|_|	|_|	|_|	__ : __	__
|_|	|_|	|_|	|_|	|_|	|_|	|_|	|_|	|_|	__ : __	__

e = return to home country; f = work abroad; g = other.
e = maternity; f = other domestic commitment; g = ill-health; h = retirement; i = other.

e = from break; f = from private practice; g = from abroad; h = other.

Annexe 2 NHS DHAs: estimated resident population at mid 1987, male and female, all ages

Area	All ages	
	Male	Female
England and Wales	24,492.8	25,750.1
England	23,115.7	24,290.9
Regional & District Health Authorities (England)		
Northern	1,498.6	1,578.2
Hartlepool	43.6	46.1
North Tees	86.3	89.5
South Tees	141.9	146.9
East Cumbria	86.0	91.7
South Cumbria	83.3	88.9
West Cumbria	67.6	69.3
Darlington	60.6	63.4
Durham	115.0	120.2
North West Durham	41.8	44.5
South West Durham	75.2	78.0
Northumberland	147.1	153.8
Gateshead	100.8	106.1
Newcastle	136.9	145.8
North Tyneside	92.2	100.6
South Tyneside	76.1	80.1
Sunderland	143.9	153.2
Yorkshire	1,754.1	1,850.5
Hull	146.5	155.4
East Yorkshire	92.6	99.6
Grimsby	78.2	80.5
Scunthorpe	94.6	99.1
Northallerton	57.3	56.6
York	129.2	134.2
Scarborough	68.9	75.5
Harrogate	64.7	70.7
Bradford	165.2	172.0
Airedale	83.8	90.1
Calderdale	94.3	100.5
Huddersfield	103.1	109.0
Dewsbury	79.8	83.9
Leeds Western	175.9	186.4
Leeds Eastern	168.4	178.3
Wakefield	70.5	73.6
Pontefract	81.3	84.9
Trent	2,285.1	2,361.2
North Derbyshire	178.1	183.9
Southern Derbyshire	259.9	267.1
Leicestershire*	434.5	444.9
North Lincolnshire	133.1	137.5
South Lincolnshire	149.1	154.9
Bassetlaw	52.5	52.4
Central Nottinghamshire	142.4	146.1
Nottingham	301.0	313.4
Barnsley	109.1	112.4
Doncaster	143.0	147.1
Rotherham	123.8	127.9
Sheffield	258.6	273.7

Area	All ages	
	Male	Female
East Anglian	986.8	1,026.8
Cambridge	135.8	137.2
Peterborough	99.3	105.7
West Suffolk	112.2	114.5
East Suffolk	157.4	163.9
Norwich	227.5	241.4
Great Yarmouth & Waveney †	95.5	102.1
West Norfolk & Wisbech	92.4	95.5
Huntingdon	66.7	66.5
North West Thames	1,703.6	1,784.6
North Bedfordshire	124.5	125.1
South Bedfordshire	137.6	138.7
North Hertfordshire	91.2	94.4
East Hertfordshire	146.7	148.8
North West Hertfordshire*	128.0	133.1
South West Hertfordshire	119.4	125.2
Barnet	146.8	159.1
Harrow	96.8	103.3
Hillingdon	112.5	118.5
Hounslow & Spelthorne	138.4	142.7
Ealing*	145.6	151.3
Brent*	125.1	131.6
Paddington & N Kensington	57.9	62.6
Riverside	133.2	150.2
North East Thames	1,830.8	1,940.7
Basildon and Thurrock	138.9	142.6
Mid Essex	142.3	147.6
North East Essex	147.6	156.8
West Essex	124.2	127.8
Southend	155.2	168.1
Barking, Havering & Brentwood	221.9	233.9
Hampstead	51.3	58.5
Bloomsbury †	60.5	68.3
Islington	81.1	87.6
City and Hackney	93.1	99.0
Newham	100.3	106.2
Tower Hamlets	79.5	79.4
Enfield	126.0	135.5
Haringey	94.5	99.2
Redbridge	111.2	118.9
Waltham Forest	103.2	111.4
South East Thames	1,750.1	1,885.4
Brighton	140.9	158.1
Eastbourne	106.7	125.8
Hastings	76.8	89.8
South East Kent	129.1	137.5
Canterbury & Thanet	144.1	158.8
Dartford & Gravesham	108.5	111.1
Maidstone	97.6	99.5
Medway †	162.0	166.6
Tunbridge Wells	94.4	101.4
Bexley	107.7	112.9
Greenwich	103.8	112.8
Bromley	145.3	152.9
West Lambeth	79.1	82.6
Camberwell	102.0	110.3
Lewisham & N Southwark	152.1	165.5

* no reply received
† reply received too late for inclusion

Area	All ages	
	Male	Female
South West Thames	1,428.5	1,531.1
North West Surrey	101.2	105.2
West Surrey & N E Hants	137.3	137.8
South West Surrey	87.7	93.7
Mid Surrey *	79.0	86.2
East Surrey	88.3	94.5
Chichester	84.6	95.5
Mid Downs	136.0	140.3
Worthing	111.0	132.5
Croydon	156.6	162.6
Kingston & Esher	85.0	90.9
Richmond, Twickenham & Roehampton	110.1	121.8
Wandsworth	92.4	96.9
Merton & Sutton	159.4	173.2
Wessex	1,416.7	1,488.9
East Dorset	211.5	236.6
West Dorset	97.0	103.5
Portsmouth & S E Hants	261.9	267.7
Southampton & S W Hants	205.3	213.5
Winchester	104.4	106.1
Basingstoke & N Hants	107.3	109.8
Salisbury	59.4	61.7
Swindon	112.7	117.5
Bath	196.9	205.8
Isle of Wight	60.3	66.6
Oxford	1,242.5	1,259.4
East Berkshire	178.7	181.0
West Berkshire	226.7	225.0
Aylesbury Vale	71.5	72.9
Wycombe	132.8	137.0
Milton Keynes	85.3	85.5
Kettering	124.6	130.4
Northampton	151.3	155.5
Oxfordshire	271.6	272.1
South Western	1,547.8	1,657.8
Bristol & Weston	176.4	190.8
Frenchay	107.6	113.0
Southmead	114.3	118.1
Cornwall & Scilly Isles	216.9	236.3
Exeter	146.8	159.4
North Devon	65.2	68.2
Plymouth	162.1	167.8
Torbay *	112.7	127.8
Cheltenham & District	101.1	109.5
Gloucester .	151.6	160.0
Somerset	193.1	206.9

Area	All ages	
	Male	Female
West Midlands	2,564.2	2,633.4
Bromsgrove & Redditch	82.9	84.0
Herefordshire	77.0	79.0
Kidderminster & District	49.6	52.1
Worcester & District	117.2	123.3
Shropshire	195.8	200.7
Mid Staffordshire	154.5	156.8
North Staffordshire	226.2	234.8
South East Staffordshire	126.8	128.4
Rugby	42.6	42.7
North Warwickshire	86.1	87.9
South Warwickshire	110.0	115.0
Central Birmingham	89.8	90.9
East Birmingham	98.7	98.9
North Birmingham	80.5	83.2
South Birmingham	120.6	125.7
West Birmingham	103.8	106.1
Coventry	153.3	155.6
Dudley	149.5	153.2
Sandwell	145.8	152.6
Solihull	99.8	104.1
Walsall	129.9	131.9
Wolverhampton	123.9	126.6
Mersey	1,166.6	1,242.1
Chester	85.7	91.3
Crewe	121.8	126.0
Halton	70.5	72.6
Macclesfield	87.1	92.2
Warrington	91.6	93.8
Liverpool	229.4	246.6
St Helens & Knowsley	169.8	178.9
Southport & Formby	55.7	63.1
South Sefton	85.9	92.7
Wirral	169.2	184.9
North Western	1,940.2	2,050.9
Lancaster	62.8	67.6
Blackpool, Wyre & Fylde	150.1	168.7
Preston	61.4	65.3
Blackburn, Hyndburn & Ribble Valley	131.2	137.4
Burnley, Pendle & Rossendale *	111.2	116.6
West Lancashire	52.0	54.7
Chorley & South Ribble	95.9	98.8
Bolton	127.9	134.4
Bury	84.4	89.3
North Manchester	70.1	72.8
Central Manchester	63.9	61.1
South Manchester	87.1	95.0
Oldham †	107.1	112.4
Rochdale	104.8	109.4
Salford *	115.7	122.0
Stockport	140.6	150.4
Tameside & Glossop	119.4	126.3
Trafford	104.2	112.0
Wigan	150.5	156.7

Area	All ages	
	Male	Female
Wales	**1,377.1**	**1,459.2**
District Health Authorities & Management Units (Wales)		
Clwyd	194.6	208.3
North Clwyd	82.3	91.4
South Clwyd	112.3	116.9
East Dyfed *	112.3	119.6
Ceredigion	31.5	33.8
Carmarthen-Dinefwr	34.7	35.9
Llanelli-Dinefwr	46.1	49.8
South Pembrokeshire	53.7	57.7
Gwent *	216.5	226.6
North Gwent Hospitals	59.6	61.9
Pontypool & W Gwent Hospitals	73.5	77.2
Newport & Chepstow Hospitals	83.4	87.5
Gwynedd	113.7	122.6
Anglesey	34.3	35.9
Meirionnydd	15.0	16.4
Aberconwy	25.2	28.3
Arfon	26.6	28.0
Dwyfor	12.7	14.0
Mid Glamorgan	260.9	273.8
Ogwr	66.7	69.1
Taff-Ely	46.4	47.3
Rhondda	37.4	39.7
Merthyr Cynon	59.7	63.7
Rhymney	50.8	54.0
Powys	56.2	57.1
Montgomery	25.0	25.6
Brecknock & Radnor	31.2	31.5
South Glamorgan	193.8	205.7
West Glamorgan	175.3	187.9
East District Hospitals	55.0	60.0
N & W District Hospitals	120.3	127.9
Scotland	**2,470.6**	**2,641.5**

Scotland: no reply received from Orkney, Shetland, Western Isle; reply received too late for inclusion from Ayrshire and Arran, Lanarkshire

Annexe 3 LASS departments: estimated resident population at mid 1987, male and female, all ages
(some may not employ OTs)

Area	All ages Male	Female
England and Wales	24,492.8	25,750.1
England	23,115.7	24,290.9
Standard Regions & Counties		
North	1,498.6	1,578.2
Tyne and Wear	550.0	585.8
Cleveland	271.9	282.6
Cumbria	237.0	249.9
Durham	292.6	306.1
Northumberland	147.1	153.8
Yorkshire and Humberside	2,388.7	2,511.6
South Yorkshire §§	634.5	661.0
West Yorkshire	998.8	1,053.6
Humberside *	411.9	434.6
North Yorkshire *	343.4	362.4
East Midlands	1,940.9	2,001.4
Derbyshire *	452.3	466.3
Leicestershire	434.5	444.9
Lincolnshire	282.2	292.3
Northamptonshire	275.9	285.9
Nottinghamshire	495.9	511.9
East Anglia	986.4	1,026.8
Cambridgeshire *	317.0	325.4
Norfolk	358.1	378.1
Suffolk	311.8	323.3
South East	11,701.9	12,386.1
Greater London ††	3,273.5	3,496.9
Inner London	1,209.4	1,302.8
Outer London	2,064.2	2,194.1
Bedfordshire *	262.1	263.8
Berkshire	370.5	370.1
Buckinghamshire *	307.4	313.8
East Sussex	324.4	373.6
Essex	743.1	778.7
Hampshire	760.0	777.0
Hertfordshire *	485.3	501.5
Isle of Wight	60.3	66.6
Kent	735.7	774.9
Oxfordshire	288.5	289.5
Surrey *	485.9	514.4
West Sussex	331.6	368.4
South West	2,215.7	2,372.7
Avon	461.1	490.1
Cornwall and Isles of Scilly	216.9	236.3
Devon *	486.8	523.2
Dorset	308.5	340.1
Gloucestershire *	252.7	269.5
Somerset	219.2	233.1
Wiltshire	270.5	280.3

Area	All ages Male	Female
West Midlands	2,564.2	2,633.4
West Midlands §	1,295.5	1,328.8
Hereford and Worcester *	326.8	338.4
Shropshire	195.8	200.7
Staffordshire *	507.5	520.0
Warwickshire	238.7	245.5
North West	3,001.6	3,184.7
Greater Manchester †	1,257.4	1,322.7
Merseyside	700.6	756.1
Cheshire	375.1	393.0
Lancashire *	668.4	712.9
Wales	1,377.1	1,459.1
Clwyd *	194.6	208.3
Dyfed	166.0	177.3
Gwent *	216.5	226.6
Gwynedd *	113.7	122.6
Mid Glamorgan	260.9	273.8
Powys	56.2	57.1
South Glamorgan	193.8	205.7
West Glamorgan	175.3	187.9
Area Aggregates		
Greater London	3,273.5	3,496.9
Inner London	1,209.4	1,302.8
Outer London	2,064.2	2,194.1
Metropolitan Districts	5,436.9	5,708.0
Principal Cities –	1,683.6	1,764.6
Others	3,753.4	3,943.4
Non-Metropolitan Districts	15,782.3	16,545.1
Cities	2,179.8	2,301.3
Industrial	3,289.7	3,414.9
With New Towns	1,134.0	1,172.7
Resort and Retirement	1,680.8	1,889.6
Mixed Urban-Rural	4,905.3	5,047.6
Remoter Largely Rural	2,592.7	2,719.0

* no reply received
No reply was received from the following districts:
† Salford, Manchester, Trafford, Stockport
‡ Barking, Bexley, Brent, Camden, Havering, Lambeth, Southwark, Tower Hamlets, Westminster
§ Wolverhampton, Sandwell, Solihull
§§ Wakefield